The
KIDNEY
STONES
Handbook

A Patient's Guide to
Hope, Cure and Prevention

Gail Golomb

Foreword by Kenneth B. Woods, M.D.

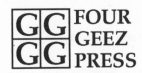

**FOUR
GEEZ
PRESS**

Roseville, CA

The author and publisher of this book are not physicians and are not licensed to give medical advice. This publication is provided to serve the reader as a supplement to professional medical guidance and treatment, not as a substitute for professional medical care. As new medical research broadens our knowledge, treatment and drug therapy adapt. The author and publisher have made every effort to ensure that information regarding medical treatment is accurate and in accordance with the standards accepted at the time of publication. Listings of centers, and clinics do not constitute a recommendation or endorsement of any individual, institution, or group.

First Edition
ISBN 0-9637068-0-2

Cover design by Grant W. Gibbs

Four Geez Press participates in the Cataloging in Publication program of the Library of Congress. However, in our opinion, the data provided us for this book by CIP does not adequately nor accurately reflect its scope and content. Therefore, we are offering our librarian/users the choice between LC's treatment and our Alternative CIP.

Publisher's Cataloging in Publication

Golomb, Gail. R.
The kidney stones handbook: a patient's guide to hope, cure and prevention / Gail Golomb; foreword by Kenneth B. Woods.
p. cm.
Includes bibliographical references and index.
ISBN 0-9637068-0-2

1. Kidney—Calculi—Popular works. I. Title.

RC916.G65 1994   616.622
                                   QBI93-1102

Golomb, Gail. R.
The kidney stones handbook: a patient's guide to hope, cure and prevention / Gail Golomb; foreword by Kenneth B. Woods.
p. cm.
Includes bibliographical references and index.
ISBN 0-9637068-0-2

1. Kidney 2. Medical Care-United States 3. Diseases related to kidney stones 4. Medical Research 5. Consumer Education 6. Stone prevention 7. Lithotripsy 8. Diet Related to Renal Stones

RC916.G65 1994   616.622

Dedication

This book is dedicated with love
to my grandmother, Nana Barfield;
to my parents, Seymour & Anne Barfield—
and to the millions out there
who have all known the pain
of kidney stones.

Acknowledgements

I would like to thank the following people who took the time to assist me with their invaluable talent in producing this book. K.D. Profitt, Medical Librarian, Sutter Resource Library, Sutter Hospitals; Gigi Politowski, Communications Director, National Kidney Foundation; Dorothy Thurmond, Medical Librarian, MLS, Guttman Library, Sacramento-El Dorado Medical Society; Robert Downing, photographer, Roseville Press-Tribune; Bob Smith, Auburn, California; Anastasia Broderick, Manager Library Services, Mosby-Year Book, Inc.; Mark Stivers, Sacramento News & Review; Audrey Scannell, aka "Mama Mac" for her advice and endless encouragement; Bettina Flores, author of "Chiquita's Cocoon" for her "you-can-do-it" comments; Rosemarie Emerson, Law Librarian; Ruth Letner, editor par excellence; Colleen Nihen, Right Angle Productions; Mark S. Samberg, M.D., urologist; Alex M. Blaine, Blaine Company Inc., Pharmaceuticals, Erlanger, Kentucky; Kenneth B. Woods, M.D., urologist; Gail Sweeney, Pacific Grove; my daughter Jennifer Golomb; my research, business partner and friend, Grant Gibbs; Jerry Barfield; and Bart the Basset who spent many hours sitting at my feet.

Dear Friend:

This book was written to give you a better understanding of your illness. Armed with the latest, most up-to-date information available on most aspects of kidney stones, including preventative measures and dietary information, you will be able to minimize the problems and pain your stones have caused you in the past.

I believe this book will substantially improve the quality of your life.

I can tell you that, as a fellow stone-sufferer, had I known the information in this book when I first experienced the shattering, ripping pain of kidney stones, I would have been less fearful and more filled with hope.

This is your book. It's to be used. Highlight, underline, write in the margins, fold corners—anything that will help you remember parts that pertain to your own condition. Enjoy.

Affectionally yours,

Gail Golomb

Table of Contents

Charts: Food sources of oxalates: calcium-oxalate stones • Low-calcium diet: calcium stones • Low calcium test diet • Low-phosphorus diet: struvite stones • Acid ash diet: calcium stones • Low purine foods: uric acid stones • Low methionine diet: cystine stones • Summary of diet principles in renal stone disease.

Foreword

Hope? Even if I have a kidney stone? That is what the title, and this book, offers to patients suffering from kidney stones.

In the last decade, health care has gone through many changes, but few rival the impact that lithotripsy has had on the treatment of kidney stones. Kidney stones can now be broken into dust without surgery in 95% of cases, sometimes under local anesthesia as an outpatient. Despite this techno-logical advance, the sufferer of kidney stones is still confronted by fear of the unknown and harbors many questions about urinary stones, their causes and prevention: Why me? How will I get rid of this stone? Will I have pain? What kind of doctor do I need?

I can think of no one better qualified to write a book for kidney stone patients than someone who has been a patient herself. Gail Golomb has been through several experiences with stones. In this book, she uses common terms that other patients can understand to explain such things as what lithotripsy means, how stones form, and what you can do to help prevent recurrent stone formation.

As a patient, Gail was eager to learn, to understand her condition and what her options for treatment were. I can honestly say there were times I secretly wished she wouldn't ask so many questions! But I recognized that any question a patient asks is a valid question worth answering, and I learned to use our visits to educate Gail. In fact, she learned so well she felt a need to share her new insight with other patients. This book is her contribution.

If you have had or now have a kidney stone, this book is for you. By providing answers to questions in layman's terms, and explaining the treatment process from start to finish, Gail will help acquaint you with modern kidney stone treatment. Your new knowledge will help calm your fears and lead to better communication between you and your doctor. By reading this book, you will be taking a giant step toward participating in treatment decisions.

Being more involved in your own care will ultimately lead to better and more satisfying results.

Kenneth B. Woods, M.D.,
Urologist

INTRODUCTION

Why I Wrote This Book

U p to 20 percent of all adult American males will have a kidney stone at some point in their life. For women, while their lifetime risk is around 5 to 10 percent, as their socioeconomic status has risen, so has their risk of forming stones.

Other published reports suggest that as many as 15 percent of all Americans have a chance of becoming a "walking gravel pit."

I was sick and tired of becoming another statistic!

Dr. Glenn M. Preminger, Associate Professor of Urology and Internal Medicine, The University of Texas Southwestern Medical Center at Dallas writes that about 50 percent of all patients experience recurrent stones within five years of the first stone.

Kidney stones have been recorded since the time of the ancient Greeks and Romans. Recent estimates show that kidney stones are at least ten times more common now than at the beginning of the century according to a study in the *Canadian Medical Association Journal*.

> Urinary stone disease also exerts a significant economic impact. Investigators have estimated that the annual direct cost of medical care for patients in the United States requiring hospitalization (including stone detection, hospital stay, and treatment) is currently costing two billion dollars a year, in addition to the significant indirect costs of time lost from work.

However, kidney stones—a prevalent source of medical disease, suffering and expense—have received little media attention. Why there is such an increase in the numbers of people who are suddenly forming kidney stones has researchers looking at many causes.

For most sufferers, kidney stones mean recurrent agony.

As a former newspaper editor, I was shocked that over a million new patients a year will develop a kidney stone and nearly 350,000 will require hospitalization. Where were the newspaper headlines screaming these statistics?

While noted in many medical journals as one of the most painful of all human conditions, kidney stones remain a silent medical disorder with severe agony.

Even patients have a difficult time finding medical articles written in simple medical terms they can understand.

Few patients have the time required to research the latest medical information which could help them understand the causes and lessen their chances of forming new stones. This information is crucial for patients who wish to become working partners with their physicians in understanding and reducing the chances of recurrent kidney stones.

I felt my own life suddenly veer "out of control" the first time I passed a kidney stone. From a desperate desire to learn more about kidney stones, my life evolved into a quest for knowledge. It continues more than three years later as I succeed in preventing new stones from forming. After extensive medical research in countless medical and public libraries, I began to understand and once again feel in charge of my health and the kidney stones which began to take over my life. I am able to ask my urologist "intelligent" questions and feel fortunate my physician is willing to take time to answer them.

As I began my own medical research, I realized the information I collected would benefit other patients with kidney stones. Thus, from a seedling of information grew a book for all kidney stone patients.

The 1987 American Kidney Fund Annual reported that in the majority of cases kidney stones can be a life-long ailment. However, most current research indicates that kidney stones, when properly treated in stone-prone patients, are preventable.

This book was written to foster an understanding of medical conditions which lead to the formation of kidney stones, the roles diet, nutrition, and lifestyle play in prevention, the importance of drug therapy and adequate fluid intake, and the options of available treatments. I believe informed patients will more likely make necessary lifestyle changes to avoid repeat kidney stones.

Since kidney stone disease is a common medical problem with many different causes, dietary restrictions and drug therapies depend on the type of stone "manufactured" by the patient.

Over the past ten years, dramatic advances in medical research have improved the quality of patient care for those with kidney stones. Shattering kidney stones with lithotripsy has given physicians new medical and surgical treatment options. This means less pain and suffering for the patient.

I have been through lithotripsy twice. Like "love," lithotripsy was "better the second time around," perhaps because I was a better, more informed patient.

Many physicians feel lithotripsy will never become obsolete because some people will continue to form stones despite dietary modifications that can control metabolic causes. One always hopes, however, that lithotripsy will be replaced as medical research advances. Understanding the roles that nutrition, lifestyle, fluid intake and medication play in the management of kidney stones is key to curbing the "stone epidemic."

Many factors can influence one's risk in developing kidney stones. These include age, heredity, occupation, social class and affluence, geographic location, climate and diet. Of these, diet—including fluid intake along with medications—are the ones most easily changed and which have the most marked effect on all urinary risk factors.

Although chronic kidney stone disease tends to run in families, the fact that your parents or siblings had kidney stones is by no means a guarantee that you will. Patient education can further decrease the risk.

If you have already formed a stone, whether your kidney stone was formed of calcium oxalate, or uric acid, or cystine, or due to struvite (infection) stones, the following chapters will detail some of the causes for each stone type and provide encouraging news on some of the latest medical advances in preventing repeat episodes of painful kidney stones.

Detailed nutrition charts, one of the most unique aspects of this book, are included to assist you in choosing foods which will not predispose you to forming new stones. Carry this book with you when you do your grocery shopping and choose wisely among a wide variety of foods which can be enjoyed for optimum health.

I wrote this book because I believe well-informed patients in partnership with their physicians can take charge of their lives and veer off the standard course of becoming repeat statistics.

I believe all that I now write. I saw positive changes take place once I realized the three emergency trips to the hospital for pain control, and two lithotripsies were my "past medical history."

With knowledge, I avoided the likely repeat of three years of non-stop kidney stone formation. Because I want to share with others, I sat down to write this book. It wasn't easy. The vital information was there...sometimes hidden deep in computer databases. Once I found it, I knew it would be invaluable to every kidney stone patient who, like me, wants to live life and every day to its fullest.

I wrote this book as a road map for your own recovery from kidney stones. This book is the only book written for kidney stone patients in the last decade containing the latest medical information, and reviewed for accuracy by two urologists.

Because I have written this book as a resource, once the patient is made aware of his own particular disorder, several references, including medical libraries, are made at the end of the book on where to obtain further medical information.

The information in this book works! Since suffering from one brutal kidney stone attack after another, after following the advice in this book, I have not "manufactured" a new stone. Now, you too can lessen your chances of living with the pain from unexpected kidney stones.

CHAPTER ONE

The Pebble That Hurts

T he sudden wave after wave of searing, ripping pain from an unexpected kidney stone knocked the wind out of me.

It was the kind of pain I soon would learn that inspires some emergency room nurses to tell their patients, both male and female, "you are going through labor pains with this one!" Kidney stone pain is known to begin suddenly and intensify over a period of 15 to 30 minutes into a steady, unbearable pain that causes nausea and vomiting.

I could handle two cesarean births, but the pain of a kidney stone was the worst I had ever felt.

> Stones that form in the kidneys and urinary tract are one of the most painful disorders to afflict human beings.
>
> **—U.S. Department of Health and Human Services**

Only a few hours earlier I thought I was developing a bladder infection (although I had not had one in a decade).

I was not ready for the hot, knife-like wrenching pain that slashed through my left side and continued down my lower abdomen. I thought if I could lie down on a heating pad, not moving at all, the pain would ease.

In addition to the pain came round after round of nausea. I became "addicted" to the toilet, vomiting until I was dehydrated. Along with the pain running up and down my left side, I felt my bladder cramp with painful spasms yet I was unable to urinate.

> I didn't know whether to stand up, sit down, lie down or die.
>
> **—Gail Golomb, Author**

My primary care physician's office would not open for another two hours. Should I go to the emergency room? I decided to wait and see.

As I counted those endless minutes that cool summer morning, I became another statistic. According to The National Kidney Foundation I was one of more than a million Americans who would develop a kidney stone that year.

As a woman, I was a relatively rare example. Stones are more common in men; four out of five patients with stones are men.

Most of these stones range in size from less than an inch to the size of a golf ball and can cause agonizing pain in the lower abdomen and back. One moment I was fine and looking forward to another hot summer day. Then, within a minute, or so it seemed, I could not stand straight. The pain was unbearable.

I should have gone immediately to a hospital emergency room. But I tried valiantly to play down the severe pain I was feeling. It was all in my head, right? And who would step in to take care of my children still sound asleep?

When Should a Person Call the Doctor?

A patient can expect a small amount of blood in the urine from minor trauma caused by the stone. Additionally, one can expect periods of intense pain.

Call your doctor or go to the emergency room if:

- Bleeding is severe and persistent with uncontrollable pain usually starting suddenly in the kidneys and moving to the groin; pain may last for minutes or hours followed by some periods of relief;

- Pain continues to be severe, unrelenting and persistent or

- Fever and chills or nausea and vomiting develop;

- Urine is cloudy or foul smelling (may be associated with infection) or

- Urine flow is blocked.

As a divorced mother, I did not want to frighten my two children. As the family's breadwinner, I had neither time nor patience to become ill. I told myself the pain was "all in my head;" I couldn't possibly be as sick as I felt.

Ha!

What I didn't know was that I had embarked on a journey of cold fear, excruciating pain, unbelievable medical expenses that would leave me on a strict budget for years, unknown procedures and tests that left me anxious and scared, and very little knowledge about the "pebble" that hurts.

The Journey

I had been sitting quietly at my computer editing a client's book on parenting. I enjoyed working in the early morning hours before my children—Gary, then 12 years-old, and Jennifer, then 9 years-old—awoke.

When the first kidney stone made its journey down my ureter, I had two options on my health care. I could use the large health maintenance organization (HMO) under which I had complete health care coverage, or consult with the friendly young internist not associated with the HMO who had come to know me well over the past seven years. I would have to pay the latter entirely out of my own pocket.

At that moment of intense pain, money had no meaning for me. I decided to go to whichever medical office answered the phone first.

I tried desperately to get through the HMO's phones that morning, but kept getting a busy signal. My pain was too intense and I had no patience to keep trying so I called the internist. They booked an appointment for me within the hour.

I was in no shape to drive a car that morning, but I took my children along as a "comfort blanket." Bewildered and scared by my pain, they could do little other than be there. Both of my children were afraid I was going to die.

Each bump in the road was like a sword through my bladder.

Once we arrived at the office, my physician immediately took an x-ray. It was the first of many to come over the years. When he returned to the examining room, he told me I was passing a kidney stone.

At that moment, it seemed the worst news he could have given me.

Visions of My Mother

The news of my kidney stone upset me tremendously. My mother, my father, my paternal grandmother and my brother had kidney stones. At times, my brother passed two every month!

I remembered how, as a young girl, I watched my mother endure horrendous pain. As I grew up, I saw the long red scar on her back from her kidney stones surgery. I remembered how I missed her when she was hospitalized.

I grew up fearing my mother's pain without understanding it. Finally, at age 38, (in my heightened state of anxiety) I was horrified to be told that my mother's pain had become my destiny.

According to the National Institute of Arthritis, Diabetes, and Digestive and Kidney Diseases of the United States Department of Health and Human Services, in the past little could be done for most patients with stones. However, "with a surprising lack of fanfare..." a noted scientist wrote recently, "recurrent renal stones have become a preventable disease."

In the past, there was treatment for only some of the rarer stone formations. Patients with the most common kinds faced the prospect of drinking large quantities of liquids and the likelihood of surgery.

The day my first stone hit me, I did not realize that medical cures, treatment, and new prevention care had dramatically advanced over the "stone age" medical management my mother received some thirty-years earlier.

Today, scientific progress has brought greater understanding of the causes and mechanisms of stone formation and far more effective clinical management of stone disease.

My internist told me that my kidney stone, due to its size, could become a life-threatening situation. He told me it was important I go to my HMO and get the care I desperately needed, as well as additional medical tests to fully evaluate my condition and hopefully prevent future stones.

"If you can't find someone to drive you, we'll call an ambulance," my doctor told me.

Learning to Ask for Help

I didn't want an ambulance, but I also didn't want to disturb my working friends. It wasn't fair to take them away from paying jobs.

I learned to change this attitude. Over the next three years, I got tired of leaving my car in the hospital lot when I was admitted as a patient and asking others to drive my car home. It was easier—and safer—for me to get a ride.

I learned to ask friends to spend the night with my children and I learned it was sometimes necessary to make a middle-of-the-night call to a friend to rush me to the emergency room. People were more than willing to lend a hand.

I developed a sense of humor that guided me through the tough times. With my first kidney stone crisis, the only person I could think of to transport me—without losing time at his work—was my former husband.

A nurse put in a call to his office, and he agreed to drive me to the hospital. During the hour I waited for him, I settled on the examining table and my doctor administered two shots for pain control. At long last I was able to lie down and relax. The hot pain in my back subsided until I arrived at the hospital. For at least one hour, I felt less nauseous than when I first arrived at my physician's office.

My former husband decided to drop off our children at home before taking me to the hospital. I tried lying down in the back seat. During the entire trip, first back to the house, and then on to the hospital, I vomited continuously into a plastic garbage can liner. Since some narcotic pain medications can cause nausea I was feeling the effects of the pain medication given to me in the doctor's office.

Symptoms of Stones

Not everyone experiences pain with kidney stones. Some have "silent" kidney stones which produce no discomfort. Many feel pain so severe that it's unforgettable. The pain may come in waves that begin in the lower back and move to the side or groin.

Typically, the patient notices aching in the back and side in the vicinity of the kidney or in the lower abdomen. Later, the pain may radiate to the groin.

If the stone is too large to pass easily, the severe constant pain continues as the muscles in the walls of the tiny ureter try to squeeze the stone along into the bladder. Sometimes patients experience a burning sensation during urination, or increased frequency of urination, or blood in the urine.

Other symptoms of stones include nausea, the presence of urinary infection accompanied by fever, vomiting, loss of appetite, and chills. The patient may find that the region of the kidney and abdomen are very tender to the touch.

Once we arrived at the hospital, my former husband gave the receptionist my medical information and health history. I spent most of the time vomiting in the restroom. When I returned to the waiting area, a wheelchair was waiting for me. The severe pain, however, prevented my relaxing long enough to sit for any length of time.

The Emergency Room

While standing up against the hospital's wall, I noticed how cool it felt against my hot back. For the next 40 minutes, until I was taken into the emergency room, I used the coolness from the wall to lessen the pain in my back. I went from sitting on the floor to standing against the wall repeatedly. Others in the emergency room must have found my antics humorous.

When my name was finally called, I was led to a gurney which became "home" for the next fourteen hours. I arrived at the hospital during the cool summer morning hours and would not leave until darkness had crept into the river city of Sacramento, California.

The hospital first placed a white patient identification band around my left wrist. From that moment on, I knew I was in serious trouble. "So this is my new reality," I thought to myself.

I was given intravenous pain medication (medication injected into a vein) and metabolic fluids to replace fluids lost during vomiting. I could absorb fluids through the intravenous (IV) hook-up, but I was given nothing to drink in case I required emergency surgery.

I began to feel the pain medication work its way through my lower back until it settled into my shoulders. Within minutes, the pain from the stone was nearly gone. At that moment, I thought it possible that life just might continue. Maybe.

The IV needle would prove helpful as the day progressed and other tests were taken.

People used to lose their kidneys before the invention of modern non-invasive treatments. The multiple operations needed to remove recurring stones often left scar tissue which could lead to complications. Eventually, some patients' kidneys stopped functioning altogether.

The emergency room physicians performed a medical evaluation, leading me through a battery of tests. It was important they know the exact location, size, and type of stone to plan further treatment. Hopefully, I would pass the stone in the emergency room so it could be retrieved and sent to a laboratory for evaluation.

If the stone proved too large to pass, I would require surgery. If there was time to spare and my condition was not life-threatening, I could wait until some later date to undergo a new stone-crushing method called lithotripsy (extracorporeal shock-wave lithotripsy or ESWL). Some medications, depending on the type of stone involved, might even dissolve the stone.

The x-ray examination in the physician's office had merely established the presence of a stone. The emergency room physicians, however, performed analyses of my blood and urine to help determine the cause (if any) of this crisis, and plan the proper course of treatment.

More x-rays of the stone were taken.

Stone in Crisis: What to Expect in the Emergency Room

In addition to x-rays, patients can usually expect an IVP (intra-venous pyelogram which uses dye to locate the stone and shows in detail the anatomy of the kidney, ureters, and bladder) and other routine procedures which are necessary to evaluate a "kidney stone in crisis." These diagnostic tests map out a plan for future prevention of recurrent kidney stone formation.

The IVP, especially for the first-time patient, can be a terrifying experience. However, when physicians who administer an IVP are understanding and take the time to reassure an anxious patient by explaining the procedure and describing what to expect, the fear diminishes.

The patient will be asked if he or she is allergic to "iodine or shellfish." Luckily, I was not—in fact, had I felt better, I would have enjoyed a lobster dinner enormously!

I felt the IVP solution travel through my vein—cold at first. Within minutes I could feel a metallic taste in my mouth. The physician explained what I might expect and stayed with me to answer any questions I had. This lessened my fear and anxiety.

After the dye was administered, x-rays which highlighted the kidneys and ureters as well as the bladder were taken.

During the day and early evening, I was given a lot of pain medication. It made me dizzy but disoriented feelings were better than managing the pain of a stone without medication.

Romancing the Stone: How to Catch a Kidney Stone

In most cases, if the stone is small, the patient needs only pain relief and instructions on how to recover the stone after it is passed. Anywhere from 70 percent to 80 percent of all stones pass when the patient urinates.

Whether one is at home or in an emergency room, I can not stress enough the importance of "catching" the stone. Several "stone catchers"—usually cone-shaped cups with cotton or mesh-like filters—are used to help strain the urine. At home, even a large aquarium strainer will do the trick! The patient urinates through these strainer cups hoping to find the stone in the filter (much like an early miner looking for gold at the bottom of the gold-pan!).

A year later, during another kidney stone crisis, when my stone snagged on my skin as I went to the bathroom, I was able to retrieve it with toilet tissue. Its sharp-sided edge felt like a rose thorn. No wonder it hurt so much!

It is important that patients ask for a mesh-like strainer before they empty their bladder in the emergency room. Sometimes in a busy emergency room, a nurse may forget to give the patient a cup or stone catcher. This has happened to me twice and the kidney stone was never found.

Catching the stone is essential so a stone analysis can be done. By identifying the stone's chemical make-up, its cause can often be determined. This, of course, helps the physician determine treatment and a prevention program.

Fourteen hours after arriving, I was finally discharged from the emergency room. Subsequent x-rays showed I had passed the stone though I did not "catch" it when emptying my bladder.

Diagnosis: They Found A Second, Even Larger Stone—Now What?

Before I left the hospital I was given even worse news: there was a second, much larger stone also in the left kidney.

In my hand, I clutched both a prescription for pain medication and an appointment for a follow-up visit with a urologist I had never met before. I was taking my first step on a long journey toward understanding what had happened to me and what, if anything, I could do to prevent such a day from ever happening again.

What I didn't know was that I would be hospitalized twice more, pass two more large kidney stones, receive lithotripsy (ESWL) twice (once in each kidney). I would greet my future reluctantly—a future I could only manage with proper nutrition, adequate fluids, medication and patient education. Fortunately, the future included some sophisticated medical advances in the management of kidney stones.

It was a future that required the team effort of myself and my urologist, a urologist who would answer *all* my questions. I no longer wanted to play the role of a faceless patient identified by a number on a white bracelet.

I was a person with a name who wanted to prevent my kidney stone scene from "playing again, Sam." I found out later how I could regain some control of my health by changing my lifestyle.

CHAPTER TWO

Are You Stone Prone?

During the 1960's, Bob Dylan sang "...everybody must get stoned...Oh, I would not feel so alone; everybody must get stoned."

While Dylan was obviously not singing about kidney stones, more than a million Americans do "get stoned" with kidney stones each year.

In addition, because renal stone formation is a chronic disease patients often form new stones within a year or two after the first is passed or removed. Eventually, nearly all patients—even single-stone formers—experience recurrence.

According to The National Institutes of Health, renal stones account for about seven to ten of every 1,000 hospital admissions in the United States. Other studies conservatively estimate there are 16 cases per 10,000 people per year.

In this country one woman in twenty and one man in seven can expect to experience the pain of kidney stones at least once before reaching the age of 70. Of all renal stones, 75 percent to 80 percent occur in men between the ages of 20 and 60. Women are one-fifth as likely as men to develop stones.

Some studies suggest that women who are not predisposed to forming kidney stones may excrete more citrate and less calcium than men, and this is perhaps a reason why men form stones more often. Other studies pinpoint lower serum testosterone levels as explaining the lower incidence in women and children.

If You've Had One Stone, You May Be Prone to Having More

The August 1992 *Mayo Clinic Health Letter* suggests that an individual is either prone to forming stones or not. No one knows why, but if you develop a stone, you may be prone to having more.

For both men and women, kidney stones usually hit at a time in their lives when social and career obligations are extremely demanding.

While researching this book, I spoke with a forty year-old man who gave up his dream of having his own family. Never married, he hoped one day to "find the right woman." However, after suffering the immense pain and fear that comes with passing one or two stones every two months for two decades, he decided to have a vasectomy. He vowed that he would never pass on to his children a family trait that might cause them to endure pain as he had.

Dr. Lynwood H. Smith of the division of nephrology at the Mayo Clinic wrote that, by the time people in the United States reach 70 years of age, 5 percent to 15 percent of the population will develop at least one urinary stone.

Kidney stones tend to occur and re-cur in specific environments and among persons with certain diseases, family and personal health histories, dietary habits, and metabolism, all of which are reflected in the urine con-tent. Knowing what these risks are enables patients predisposed to form-ing stones to avoid developing them, and to help stone-forming patients to avoid recurrences.

—Dr. Alan G. Wasserstein
Assistant Professor of Medicine
Renal Electrolyte Section of
University of Pennsylvania School
of Medicine, Philadelphia
***Consultant*, May 1986**

What is a Kidney Stone?

The makeup of a kidney stone is interesting—a hardened mineral deposit containing calcium and other chemicals. It begins as a microscopic particle and grows slowly, developing into a stone over a period of months or even years.

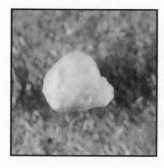

This is a magnified photograph of a calcium oxalate stone. The exterior layers are composed of calcium oxalate and the interior layer of 100 percent calcium phosphate. The stone may have origi-nated as an infection, or struvite stone, then collected calcium oxalate and grew. The author was able to pass this stone in the emergency room.

Kidney stones accumulate layers in much the same way rock candy does. The hard mass occurs when certain chemicals in the urine form crystals which then stick together. The majority of stones (nearly 80 percent) contain mainly calcium oxalate crystals.

The stone's composition helps reveal its cause and sets the stage for treatment. However, it is not unusual for a kidney stone to be composed of two or more chemicals.

Clues to the Kidney Stone Mystery

What causes stones, why 60 percent to 80 percent of stone victims are male and why this disease rarely affects children are questions scientists have tried to answer for hundreds of years. In 1985, researchers at the American Chemical Society's 190th national meeting in Chicago discussed a partial answer to the question: what causes stones? Researchers at the University of Chicago four years earlier had discovered a mechanism that appeared to keep seed crystals from forming in patients without kidney stones. Glycoprotein in their urine was found to coat microscopic seed crystals, thus preventing further deposits of calcium oxalate layers. This is encouraging information for the stone-prone!

The Chicago researchers identified a condition which made chronic stone formers different: they apparently lack an essential amino acid. In people who did not form kidney stones, an enzyme changes a precursor molecule produced by the kidney into the stone-inhibiting glycoprotein. However, according to chemist Yasushi Nakagawa, in calcium oxalate forming individuals, the enzyme responsible for making the glycoprotein either malfunctions or is present in insufficient quantities. Because some of the "inhibitor" present in these patient's urine lacks this apparently crucial amino acid, it does not block crystal growth.

Fortunately, there are ways to compensate for this diffi-culty. Patients who lack the amino acid can make dietary changes to slow the rate of any incubating stone's growth. The ultimate goal of the research, according to Nakagawa, is to discover what partially shuts down the production of this acid in the kidneys and to find ways to restore the ability to make functional crystal-growth inhibitors.

The good news is that today physicians can prescribe specific measures to prevent recurrence for most of their patients.

What Kidney Stones Look Like

Kidney stones vary in appearance. Coloration varies depending on the chemical composition. Stones composed of calcium phosphate are generally yellow or brown. Cystine stones are yellow in color. Uric acid stones range from yellow to light brown. Colors may also be affected by deposits of pigment or cellular material.

When collecting a kidney stone for analysis by the physi-cian, be on the lookout for brown, tan, gold, or black specks as well as pebbles. *These are all kidney stones.*

Stones can be rounded, jagged, or even branched.

Determining exactly what type of stone a patient has passed and the mechanism by which it formed is of utmost importance. The physician must have this information to provide appropriate preventative treatment. By conducting extensive tests, a physician can determine what metabolic disturbance caused the stone. Kidney stones are the end result of this disorder.

Because each patient is unique and the causes for the metabolic disorders vary widely, patients should work closely with their physician to determine the cause of their particular stone.

Some Common Causes of Kidney Stones

In some cases, the cause for kidney stones may be "idiopathic." In other words, there is no obvious cause. But often kidney stone formation can be traced to specific conditions.

A medical diagnosis of hypercalcemia means the cause of the stone is due to high levels of calcium in the blood, believed to be a result of diet.

More than three-quarters of all renal-stone patients form calcium oxalate stones. Approximately 40 percent of these patients have an inherited tendency to excrete excessive calcium, a condition termed either idiopathic (unknown) or benign hypercalciuria.

Many of these stones also contain another chemical: oxalate, for example. Calcium oxalate crystals may form spontaneously.

And Another Risk: High Blood Pressure

If you have high blood pressure, you may also be at risk for forming kidney stones. A medical study in the *British Medical Journal* (May 12, 1990) suggested that individuals with high blood pressure do not absorb calcium properly in the kidneys. Since high levels of calcium in the body is the most common cause of kidney stones, individuals with high blood pressure may have an increased incidence of kidney stones.

The researchers, Drs. Francesco P. Cappuccio, Pasquale Strazzullo and Mario Mancini showed that individuals with high blood pressure were twice as likely to have kidney stones in the urinary tract. This was observed after other factors were adjusted such as age, body mass, kidney function, blood urate and calcium concentrations. When only those receiving treatment for high blood pressure were considered, the risk of developing kidney stones tripled.

If you have high blood pressure and kidney stones, it's important to discuss this condition with your physician.

Kidney Stone Incidence Continues to Increase

The incidence of renal or kidney stones is on the rise. From 1952 to 1974, the frequency of kidney stones as a hospital discharge diagnosis increased by 75 percent! Some researchers feel there is an epidemic of kidney stones. This, of course, includes both first-time stones and repeaters.

The average rate of new stone formation in calcium-stone patients who have previously formed a stone is about one stone every year or two after the first is passed. Other research indicates that chances are greater than one in two that a patient will suffer another stone within five to ten years unless preventative treatment is given and/or lifestyle changes take place.

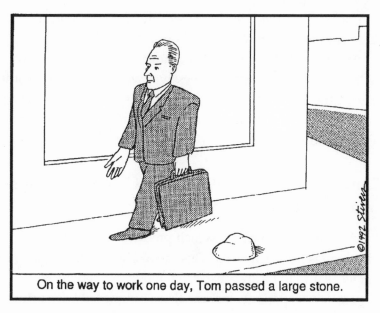

On the way to work one day, Tom passed a large stone.

Reprinted with permission; Mark Stivers, Sacramento, CA.

Are You Stone Prone?

In most cases, a combination of factors causes kidney stones. Physicians have identified several characteristics that appear to increase an individual's risk of developing a kidney stone.

The typical kidney stone sufferer is male, between 20 and 60 years of age, and has a family history that includes stone formation. A family history of stone formation does not necessarily inform the physician of the type of stone. All kinds of stones, except perhaps struvite (or infection stones), tend to run in families.

Medical conditions often play a role in stone formation. Endocrine disorders, chronic dehydration, urinary tract obstructions, recurrent infections and genetic disorders can lead to kidney stones.

Bowel disease can raise calcium oxalate levels and promote stone growth.

It is possible that without these "defects" present, some patients may be at risk for developing stones.

Anything that decreases the amount of fluid in the body, such as a low liquid intake, excessive sweating, or hot weather may set the stage for kidney stone formation. Some regions of the United States are known as "kidney stone belts" because of higher incidence apparently due to hot, dry climate.

Conditions Which May Form Calcium Stones— Genetic Disorders and Others

One medical condition which produces calcium stone formation is hypercalciuria. This metabolic disorder causes too much calcium to be absorbed from foods the patient eats. Hypercalciuria patients include those diagnosed with primary hyperparathyroidism. Other causes include toxic levels of vitamin A or D; excessive dietary protein, sodium or calcium.

Patients who are immobilized (from paralysis or prolonged bed rest) may have more calcium in the urine and thereby increased odds for forming a kidney stone.

Certain drugs (such as furosemide, steroids, or antacids) may also put some patients at risk for hypercalciuria.

Antacids, with or without calcium, can cause stone formation since they cause phosphate depletion that can increase urine calcium excretion.

Another medical condition, hyperoxaluria, may be caused by excessive oxalate or insufficient calcium in diet. Hyperoxaluria may be caused by a pyridoxine deficiency or vitamin C abuse.

Excessive uric acid in one's diet may cause another stone forming condition called hyperuricosuria. Patients with gout also have excessive uric acid and thus may be prone to forming stones.

Any of these conditions can be detected by a urologist through specific blood and urine tests.

Water! Water! Water! And Then More!

If a patient prone to forming kidney stones lives in a hot climate and perspires heavily, large amounts of fluids may be lost. If this water is not replaced, the urine will become concentrated with solute (a substance that can be dissolved in liquid). The minerals the urine contains (such as calcium) which normally are dissolved, tend to solidify into anything from gravel to full-blown stones.

When urine is concentrated with solute, crystals can separate and become the core of a future kidney stone.

Conditions Which Block the Flow of Urine

Functioning kidneys, like a well-oiled luxury car, can be impaired by a variety of conditions. These conditions include inflammatory and degenerative disease; chronic diseases (such as hypertension, diabetes mellitus and gout); environmental agents (such as insecticides, solvents, toxic substances), some medications and trauma.

Urinary Tract Infections

Kidney stones (renal calculi) and urinary tract infections all affect the structure and function of the kidneys. A common infection is called cystitis, an inflammation of the bladder which is prevalent in young women. The condition is called "recurrent" UTI (urinary tract infection) if three or more bouts are experienced in a year. Untreated urinary tract infections may also lead to kidney stones.

And the Vitamin C Question

Many people believe that megadoses of vitamin C can cure everything from the common cold to cancer. A recent study suggests that the "wonder vitamin" may not be so wonderful for people at risk for developing kidney stones.

High doses of vitamin C (above 0.5 or 1.0 g per day) may promote stone formation.

The May 1992 *Journal of Urology* reported that urologists at the Long Island Jewish Medical Center gave 15 patients doses of vitamin C that ranged from 100 to 2,000 milligrams, and then checked their urine for oxalate. Excess vitamin C was found in the urine of patients taking 500 milligrams or more.

This study is important. It was known from previous studies that vitamin C turns into oxalate when exposed to air.

Some doctors argued that previous researchers hadn't taken adequate precautions to preserve the urine, thus exposing the vitamin C to air. The Long Island study used patients with a catheter placed right inside their kidney, thus reducing the risk of exposure to air.

The *Journal of Urology* reports that while this study will not settle the argument about the benefits of vitamin C supplements, it may convince those with a history of kidney stones to stick to a daily glass of orange juice.

One patient interviewed for this book, a big, burly home builder who lives in California's Sierra foothills, reported that he used to consume large amounts of Vitamin C. "I never had a cold in my life. I had kidney stones, but I never had a cold," he said.

His physician suggested that he stay away from excessive amounts of Vitamin C. "Now, I get colds all the time, but I sure as heck haven't had a stone in 10 years!" he exclaimed.

The Very Latest on Orange Juice

In December 1993, *Prevention Magazine* along with several other newspapers published a study suggesting an intriguing possibility: orange juice, naturally rich in both potassium and citrate, may be effective for preventing conditions leading to at least two types of kidney stones—those containing mostly uric acid or calcium phosphate. The pilot study doesn't reveal what orange juice's actual effect on stone formation is. The research also suggests that if orange juice does work, it's not likely to work as well for preventing calcium-oxalate stones. The original study was published in *Journal of Urology*, June 1993.

Avoiding the Substances Which Form Stones

People with kidney stones must avoid foods rich in the organic substances contributing to their stones. These organic substances can originate or develop into stones by providing the core or nucleus (nidus) which acts as a seed crystal in a stone just beginning.

Sources of such organic materials include bacteria masses from recurrent urinary infections, renal tissue that has sloughed off from the urinary tract, and possibly calcified plaques.

A Diet of Affluence: You Are What You Eat

The Western diet is suspect as a predisposing factor in the development of *chronic renal failure*. Research indicates that diet can lead to the formation of kidney stones. A diet including excess protein may burden our kidneys—which were not designed to handle a steady diet of protein-rich foods.

Diet can be a "can of worms"—not those necessarily found on fresh vegetables!

Researchers have found a number of possible links between diet and stone formation. Data obtained in a variety of countries including Germany and Austria suggest a strong correlation between affluence and kidney stones.

During the twentieth century in Great Britain, Germany, Italy and Norway, the incidence of clinical stone disease was closely correlated with the political and economic circumstances in each society, according to Dr. Stanley Goldfarb, Co-chief of the Renal-Electrolyte Section at the University of Pennsylvania medical school.

Studies by Dr. Goldfarb suggest that patients with recurrent kidney stones are more sensitive to the chemicals found in proteins.

In populations whose intake of dietary protein is reduced or absent, such as vegetarians, the risk of kidney stone disease is markedly reduced.

In studies carried out in Great Britain, the prevalence of stone formation in a group of vegetarians was one-third that of the general population. Dr. Goldfarb reports that vegetarians, typically members of England's upper social classes, form stones at approximately one-eighth the rate of predictions for the general population.

Even though eating vegetables means some oxalate rich food may be consumed, vegetarianism seems to provide a protective effect.

> Adequate water intake is sufficient to prevent recurrence in over 60 percent of all cases.
>
> — Guy W. Leadbetter, M.D., and
> Jay Y. Gillenwater, M.D.
> *The Journal of The American Medical Association,*
> June 19, 1991

Whether modifying dietary protein intake will produce a long-lasting remission from recurrent kidney stones remains to be shown. While research continues, a wise patient will avoid diets rich in the substances which contributed to their stone.

It's important to note, however, that restricting dietary calcium may do more harm than good if it results in increased urinary oxalate excretion. A small increase in such urine oxalate excretion could enhance stone formation more than would a large increase in urinary calcium excretion. Dietary calcium and oxalate levels continue to be studied and patients will read contradicting results. It's important to ask the urologist what he or she suggests when it comes to restricting or increasing calcium.

Other Metabolic Reasons

Metabolic disorders that prevent the body from effectively breaking down certain minerals may predispose some people to stone formation.

A stone can form only when urine is supersaturated with stone-causing crystals. Supersaturation means that the concentration of a stone forming salt, such as calcium oxalate, exceeds its solubility in urine.

This is similar to school experiments where salt is dissolved in water. While small amounts will dissolve, greater amounts will settle at the bottom of the glass.

> Urine of most normal people is supersaturated with respect to calcium oxalate, so—in principle—all people can form such stone.
>
> **—National Institutes of Health Consensus Development Conference Statement March 30, 1988**

> Renal calculi are common; the lifetime risk for men in North America is about 20 percent, and the likelihood of a recurrence after the first stone is 50 percent at five years. When a patient has stone disease start at age 25 compared with age 45, or a positive family history, the likelihood of the recurrence of stones is approximately doubled.
>
> **—Dr. Roger A. L. Sutton**
> ***The Western Journal of Medicine***
> **September 1991**

Diagnosis: Absorptive Hypercalciuria

Absorptive hypercalciuria is a condition in which a person's body absorbs calcium from food at an abnormally high rate, and empties the excess calcium through the bloodstream and kidneys into the urine. This high level of urinary calcium sometimes may cause crystals of calcium oxalate or calcium phosphate to form and grow in the kidneys or urinary tract.

In some cases, a person may habitually eat too much food that is high in calcium, thus resulting in excessive calcium being passed through the kidneys. Normally, urine contains chemical substances that inhibit the formation of crystals. These inhibitors do not seem to work for everyone, however, and some people form stones even though their urine does not show abnormally high levels of calcium.

Diagnosis: Hyperuricosuria—Uric Acid Stones

Another cause of stone formation is hyperuricosuria (a disorder of uric acid metabolism prevalent in patients with gout). Patients who are hyperuricemic may find the prescription drug allopurinol useful. Other patients can achieve alkalinization of their urine with Shohl's solution or sodium bicarbonate under the direction of their physician. Urine pH should be checked intermittently to ensure a pH higher than 7.0.

As many as 50 percent of patients with gout also have hyperuricemia which predisposes them to forming uric acid stones. There are patients without gout who pass uric acid stones.

Diagnosis: Calcium Stones and Hyperparathyroidism

Overactive parathyroid glands, or excessive consumption of vitamin D may lead to calcium stones. Large amounts of vitamin D may cause increased calcium absorption from the intestine as well as increased calcium withdrawal from the bones.

A tumor of the parathyroid glands (parathyroid adenoma), or even leukemia may cause kidney stones. The parathyroid adenoma is a benign tumor that produces an overabundance of parathyroid hormones. These hormones release calcium out of the bones and into the urine where it then forms stones. This disorder is diagnosed by a simple blood test.

Stones and the Environment

Other factors that may play a role in the formation of kidney stones include the availability of drinking water, the type and amount of trace elements in drinking water and food, and the person's occupation.

Drs. Walter M. O'Brien, James E. Rotolo and John J. Pahira of Georgetown University Hospital reported that the frequency of stones increased in certain geographic areas. According to their published article in *AFP*, November 1987, within the United States the areas of highest incidence of kidney stones are the Northwest, the Southeast, and the Southwest.

Hot weather which causes a patient to perspire seems to be directly related to an increased frequency of kidney stone formation. In the southeastern United States, for example, urinary stones are greatest from June through September. In western Australia, the incidence is highest from December through March, the Australian summer.

The Stone Belt of the United States—
And the Winner is:

It is interesting to note that in the United States the "kidney stone belt" is centered in the Carolinas. Tennessee has the highest reported prevalence of kidney stones of any other population studied.

A fascinating study on risk factors in a regional area was reported by Michael J. Thun and Susan Schober in *The American Journal of Public Health*, May 1991. Thun and Schober studied four groups of workers in eastern Tennessee. They found that several characteristics were associated with workers who tended to form stones: greater weight, less frequent consumption of moonshine liquor, and higher prevalence of kidney stones and urinary infections in their families. The most important risk factors were higher age (24 percent risk by age 60), family history of stones, and the concentration of calcium oxalate in the urine.

The researchers, however, found that additional population-based data, rather than data from hospital discharge records, is needed to accurately determine the prevalence and cause of kidney stones in males living in the Southeast.

If patients are not treated after the occurrence of their first stone, additional stones will form in more than 50 percent of them.

—Dr. Lynwood H. Smith
Division of Nephrology
Mayo Clinic

Dr. Glenn M. Preminger, urologist at the University of Texas Southwestern Medical Center in Dallas writes that "unless we treat the cause, the patient will form new stones."

Kidney stones can damage the kidney. Some patients on dialysis (a process in which toxic substances, such as blood, are separated from the body and "cleansed" through a machine) have reported that their troubles began with kidney stones. The damage a stone may cause depends on its location in the kidney or urinary tract. If the stone settles in a crucial area of the kidney or urinary tract, it will cause more damage or problems than in other areas of the kidney. Infections associated with kidney stones may also lead to kidney damage if left untreated.

The bottom line for patients who are stone prone is that there is hope, and in many cases long-term prevention. In the next chapter I will identify specific types of stones and the latest medical advances in preventing them.

CHAPTER THREE

Different Types of Stones— Calcium Oxalate, Struvite, Uric Acid and Cystine

N ot all stones are as famous as the rock group "The Rolling Stones."

Kidney stones are neither famous nor fun.

What is known is that this ancient health problem tormented numerous famous historical figures including Benjamin Franklin, Frances Bacon, Isaac Newton, Peter the Great, and Louis XIV.

Today's television personalities Harry Smith, co-host for CBS' *This Morning* and Andy Rooney of CBS' *60 Minutes* have both been plagued with kidney stones. Rooney bemoaned the fact that his kidney stone cost him a total of $11,360.83 after his two-day and three-night hospital stay for what he called "the procedure."

> Scientists have found evidence of the occurrence of stones in an Egyptian mummy, dating about 4,800 B.C.
>
> **—U.S. Department of Health and Human Services**

Not all stones look like pebbles found on the beach. A stone may be as small as a grain of sand or as large as a golf ball. Smooth, round stones may pass easily when they are small, but large ones often lead to complications.

Fortunately, about 80 percent of kidney stones pass spontaneously in the urine, usually within 48 hours of an acute attack.

However, stones with sharp jagged edges often lodge inside the kidney, ureter, or at the outlet of the bladder. In addition to pain, complications from kidney stones include infection, urinary tract obstruction and even loss of kidney function if not relieved. Infection which develops in a blocked upper urinary tract is particularly dangerous and can cause irreversible kidney and ureteral damage within days.

Struvite (also known as staghorn or infection stones), can fill the entire kidney, and are often too large to pass naturally.

Everything You Wanted to Know—But Were Afraid to Ask—About the Urinary System

A basic, simple introduction to the urinary system is important in understanding how and why kidney stones develop.

The urinary system consists of two kidneys, two "drainage tubes" called ureters, and the urethra (the tube through which urine flows from the bladder to outside the body). The kidneys, located below the ribs toward the middle of the back,

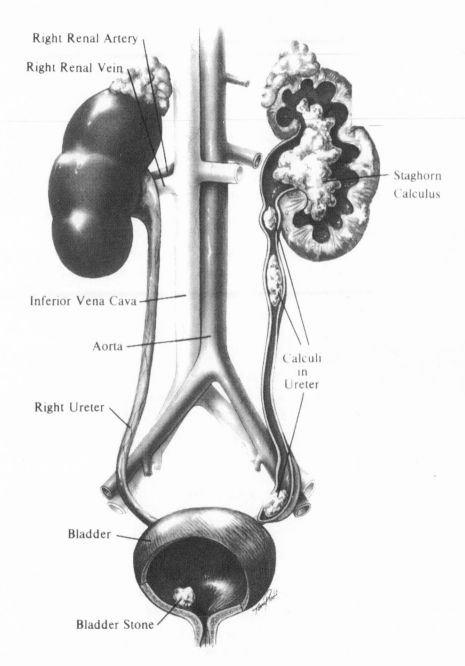

Right Renal Artery

Right Renal Vein

Staghorn Calculus

Inferior Vena Cava

Aorta

Calculi in Ureter

Right Ureter

Bladder

Bladder Stone

Illustration courtesy of Blaine Company Inc., Pharmaceuticals; Erlanger, Kentucky.

serve as chemical "filters" for the body. The ureters measure up to nine inches and connect the kidneys to the bladder in the lower abdomen. The urethra measures only about 1 1/2 inches in a woman, but up to 8 inches in a man.

The bladder, a muscular, balloon-like bag stores the urine. A man's full bladder may hold as much as 1.2 pints. A woman's is somewhat less.

Kidneys are bean-shaped systems which contain about a million filter units each. They regulate the body fluids and remove waste products by filtering various minerals, substances and water from the blood stream and excreting them as urine.

Normally, if these substances are not needed, they flow out of the body in the urine. However, the trouble begins when there is too much of a substance—such as calcium—and not enough fluid to wash it out.

Healthy kidneys screen blood throughout the day and night, working to separate chemicals from everything a person eats and drinks. Healthy kidneys filter well and release the dissolved chemicals the body doesn't need through the urine.

Micturition (urination) occurs upon relaxation of the sphincter between bladder and urethra.

From the kidneys via ureter to bladder via urethra—these are the passages from which a kidney stone travels. Since the tubes are narrow, it is no wonder that kidney stones may cause severe pain.

How Kidney Stones Form

I imagine the early formation of a kidney stone as a mini-creation. Beginning with microscopic nuclei and mixing in organic material (in the case of kidney stones—crystals), a rock kept forming. When I'm in a stone crisis, it feels as if I'm passing the entire Earth!

When a mineral such as calcium combines with a substance such as oxalate in a concentration too dense to dissolve, it can form a small crystal that will attract another, then another and so on until—voila! a kidney stone develops.

Kidney stones either remain in the kidney or break loose from its lining and move to other parts of the urinary system. These are sometimes referred to as "urinary stones."

At this point, however, patients usually begin to call their kidney stone the "Pebble from Hell." As the stone travels, it distends the ureter's narrow diameter and gouges its walls. Patients will often find bloody urine as the stone edges down—and hopefully, out!

Sometimes smaller stones pass through the ureters and lodge in the bladder where they enlarge, or stones may originate in the bladder. In either case, these are referred to as "bladder stones."

It's important to remember that whenever they occur and whatever they consist of, stones produced within the urinary system are not the disease itself, but are the end product of a disease process.

> Patients with first-time stones should receive advice on non-specific measures for preventing future stones; those with stone recurrence should undergo evaluation to identify specific metabolic abnormalities that may be corrected by medical therapy.
>
> **James E. Lingeman, M.D.,**
> **Glenn M. Preminger, M.D.,**
> **David M. Wilson, M.D.**
> ***Patient Care*, September 30, 1990**

Each individual disorder requires individualized therapy on the recommendation of the patient's physician—including dietary modifications, medications and the most important advice: to drink large amounts of water as I have previously written.

■ Calcium Oxalate Stones

The most common stones are made of calcium oxalate, a hard salt compound, or calcium oxalate mixed with calcium phosphate. Seventy to eighty percent of kidney stones are made of these calcium salts. Until recently, the causes of calcium oxalate stones could not be precisely identified. Consequently, prevention measures were frequently non-existent or unsuccessful.

However, it is now possible to identify the metabolic reasons of calcium oxalate stone formation and prescribe preventative measures against recurrence in 80 percent of all patients.

Nearly 40 percent of patients with these kind of stones have an inherited tendency to excrete excessive calcium. This condition is sometimes called idiopathic (cause unknown) hypercalciuria. In this condition, the urine is normally super-saturated with crystalized elements for no known reason. Apparently in the case of individuals who form such stones there is a lack of normal urine substances which prevent masses of crystals from forming.

Patients with calcium oxalate stones are usually advised to avoid foods with high oxalate content, including spinach, chocolate, tea, cola, rhubarb, parsley, peanuts, pecans, citrus fruits, amaranth, sesame seeds and Halva (see Chapter Five on Nutrition for a detailed list of high oxalate foods).

In some cases, patients should also avoid foods fortified with vitamin D and antacids which have a calcium base.

Drinking large amounts of milk and using medications for peptic ulcers can contribute to excess calcium. Thus, cutting down on milk products and avoiding such calcium-based medications is recommended.

The age-old treatment of increasing the patient's daily consumption of liquids (primarily water) is a worthwhile preventive measure regardless of the type of stones involved.

Although medications can't dissolve calcium oxalate stones, they can often help prevent them.

Additionally, a low-calcium diet of about 400 mg daily is usually given. This amount is half of an average adult intake of 800 mg. This lower level is achieved mainly by removal of milk and dairy products. Other calcium food sources affected are leafy vegetables and whole grains.

If the stone is calcium phosphate, phosphorus foods would also be reduced. This can be accomplished mainly by removal of milk and dairy products.

Sometimes a test diet of 200 mg. calcium (see Chapter Five on Nutrition) may be used to rule out hyperparathyroidism as a factor.

Since calcium stones have an alkaline chemistry, an acid ash diet may also be used to create an urinary environment less conducive to the formation of basic stone elements. (The classification of food groups is based on the pH of the metabolic ash produced). An acid ash diet would increase the amount of meat, grains, eggs, and cheese. It would limit the amount of vegetables, milk, and fruits.

Recent studies have shown vitamin B6 and magnesium supplements help reduce oxalate levels and inhibit stone formation in some people.

Patients with calcium oxalate stones should also avoid taking vitamin C supplements because about one-half of ingested ascorbae is converted to oxalic acid. More studies of patients with renal stones are needed before precise conclusions can be reached regarding vitamin C.

■ Uric Acid Stones

Uric acid stones account for about 20 percent of the total incidence of renal stones. Men are more prone to this type of stone which may also result in gout. Patients will need to cut down on grapes, instant coffee, berries, citrus fruits, juices, and certain vegetables.

Uric acid crystals can provide surfaces in which calcium and oxalate anchor themselves in patterns that provide a foundation for additional formation of calcium oxalate crystals.

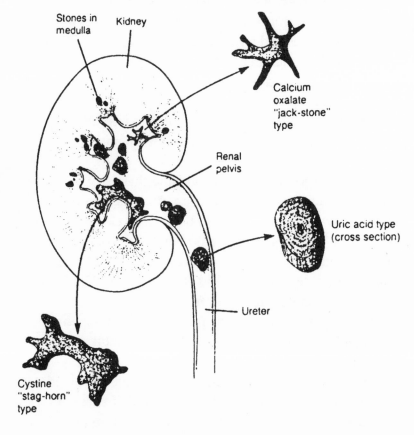

Stones in kidney and ureter.

Reprinted with permission from Times Mirror Mosby College Publishing, *Nutrition & Diet Therapy* by Sue Rodwell Williams, Ph.D., M.P.H., R.D., 5th Edition, 1985.

Hyperuricosuria can result from eating an excessive amount of meat, fish or poultry, and almost always can be controlled if the patient changes his diet.

Other foods to avoid include alcohol, sardines, anchovies, herring and organ meats such as liver.

Patients who have had a portion of their colon removed can become more acidic and also tend to dehydrate, and thus are prone to stone formation.

■ Allopurinol and Uric Acid Stones

For those patients who find it difficult to change their dietary habits, stone formation may be prevented through use of a drug called allopurinol (some commonly used brand names in the United States are Lopurin and Zyloprim) all of which reduce production of uric acid.

Allopurinol works by causing less uric acid to be produced by the body. It is available only with a doctor's prescription.

To help prevent kidney stones while taking allopurinol, adults should drink at least 10 to 12 full glasses (8 ounces each) of fluids each day unless otherwise directed by the physician.

The physician should check the patient's progress at regular visits. A blood test may be needed to make sure that this medicine is working properly and is not causing unwanted effects.

Drinking too much alcohol may increase the amount of uric acid in the blood and lessen the effects of allopurinol.

Also, taking too much vitamin C may make the urine more acidic and increase the possibility of kidney stones forming while the patient is taking allopurinol. It's important to check with the physician before taking vitamin C while taking allopurinol.

Bicarbonate, or similar drugs, may dissolve this type of stone.

Gout, a disorder of purine metabolism which is associated with arthritis, may also cause hyperuricemia, hyperuricosuria, and uric acid stones. Gout requires specific drug treatment.

Citrate drugs are sometimes also used along with other medicines to help treat kidney stones that may occur with gout.

The Nutrition Chapter in this book has an extensive list of foods which will discourage formation of uric acid stones.

■ Struvite or Infection Stones

Struvite, or infection, stones account for about 10 percent of all kidney stones. Struvite stones are composed of a simple compound—magnesium ammonium phosphate and carbonate apatite. They are also called "urease stones" and "triple-phosphate stones."

Struvite stones form because certain bacteria that grow in the urine produce ammonia, thus making the urine alkaline. This creates a wonderful condition for these stones to form.

They can be very difficult stones to treat because they often result from urinary tract infections. They can recur even after the stones have been removed. This type of stone can fill the entire inside of the kidney, spreading into the smallest passages, blocking drainage of urine, and resulting in severe kidney damage.

Struvite stones occur mainly due to infection with a certain type of urea-splitting bacteria (for example, *Proteus mirabilis* species which is identified in 72 percent of bacterial isolates) that tend to flourish and invade the kidney following a course of antibiotic therapy. More than 45 different micro-organisms produce urease. Thus, the urinary pH becomes alkaline, and in the ammonia-rich environment struvite forms large, staghorn calculi. Surgical removal is usually indicated.

Normally, women are affected more often with infection stones than men because of their increased susceptibility of urinary infections. Antibiotics are ineffective because they cannot penetrate the stone; usually a urologist needs to remove the stones surgically. At this time, lithotripsy (ESWL) can be used to "smash" struvite stones small enough to pass through the urine.

Recent research has found an agent called acetohydroxamic acid (AHA), an inhibitor of the chemical action caused by the invading bacteria, which can be used to effectively retard struvite stone formation.

There are several other urease inhibiting drugs which a physician may choose in the prevention of infection stones as well.

If you have an infection stone, your doctor may prescribe antibiotics before and after removing your stone. Prevention may include antibiotics for several months or even years.

Other disorders which may lead to struvite stones include primary gout, severe dehydration, chronic diarrheal states, and chemotherapy.

Additionally, anatomical abnormalities may need to be corrected to prevent further infection stones from forming.

Drs. Seth P. Lerner, Malachy J. Gleeson and Donald P. Griffith in *The Journal of Urology*, March 1989 reported that diet and prescription medications offer only the hope of slowing growth and/or recurrence in patients with chronic urease-producing bacteriuria. They also wrote that extreme dietary restriction of protein and magnesium offer preventative measures.

The *Mayo Clinic Health Letter* suggests that anyone prone to forming a kidney stone can develop a struvite stone. If a stone is developing in the kidney, the presence of the ammonia-producing bacteria can transform it into a struvite stone.

■ Cystine Stones

Another type of stone occurs in patients with a relatively rare inherited defect resulting in cystinuria. About 1 percent of the total stones produced are cystine. In this disorder, the amino acid—cystine—overloads the urine where it then crystallizes and forms stones. This is a heredity disorder in which the kidney fails to reabsorb cystine, thus putting patients at risk for forming cystine stones.

Prevention of cystine stones is difficult because there is no definitive treatment. Since this disorder is of a genetic origin, patients are characterized by early age onset and a positive family history. This is one of the most common metabolic disorders associated with renal stones before puberty.

Patients are advised to limit high-methionine foods (fish is the most common) which increases the production of cystine. A low-methionine diet is listed in the Nutrition Chapter.

The main therapy consists of drinking enough water to dissolve the cystine that escapes into the urine each day. This therapy can be difficult because cystine is eliminated continuously, and the patient may be required to drink over a gallon of water every 24 hours. At night, about a third of a gallon of water may be consumed on this regimen, thus filling the bladder repeatedly and interfering with sleep.

Sometimes when these stones cannot be controlled through increased fluid consumption, the drug penicillamine is administered to make cystine more soluble. This approach is always used cautiously, however, because patients may have severe allergic reactions to this drug.

A new Japanese-made drug marketed here under the name Thiola has been found effective in controlling the formation of cystine stones.

Bicarbonate, or similar drugs, dissolves cystine stones.

With all cases of kidney stones, the patient's diet, and appropriate medication(s) should be established by a physician trained in the treatment of kidney stones and urinary tract infections. Regardless of the number of stones a patient has passed, most of the diagnostic work can be done in the physician's office.

The most basic step to take in the prevention of kidney stones is to analyze the stone's composition. However, the patient must "catch" the stone. Several different ways of "catching" a stone are discussed in the book.

Patients who continue to form stones even after following established preventative measures will be glad to know that a non-surgical treatment exists for stone removal. This is especially important for people in certain working situations. You wouldn't want your airline pilot to suddenly go through a stone crisis on a nonstop flight to Australia!

A patient's guide to lithotripsy is found in the next chapter.

CHAPTER FOUR

Lithotripsy: The Patient's Guide to Non-Surgical Kidney Stone Removal

I f you've experienced the pain of a kidney stone, you know why some individuals simply must be stone free. Some professionals can not afford to, for the safety of others, experience an incapacitating attack on the job. A surgeon is a classic example. An airline pilot is another. With a little imagination, you can think of others who require prompt attention and quick relief if kidney stones were to develop.

In the past, people used to lose their kidneys before the invention of modern non-invasive treatments because the multiple operations needed to remove recurring stones caused scar tissue which led to complications and eventually, kidneys which stopped functioning. Today's technology includes modern laser, ultrasonic and fiber optic advances.

Calcium oxalate stones—including cystine stones—are tough but not as tough as they're cracked up to be. Lithotripsy can usually handle stones the size of a nickel, but larger stones may need many strong shock waves or several sessions of lithotripsy.

The procedure which shatters kidney stones into fragments so small they can pass through the ureter and the bladder where they finally leave the body via the urethra when the patient urinates is called lithotripsy or ESWL (extracorporeal shock wave lithotripsy).

Lithotripsy comes from the Greek word meaning "stone crushing." And it does indeed crush many kidney stones.

Lithotripsy, though not destined to be the "shock heard around the world," at least has made giant waves in reducing human suffering and revolutionizing the treatment of kidney stones.

Over a decade ago, the Dornier HM3 made medical headlines as the first of several lithotripters to shatter kidney stones non-invasively.

At that time, in the October 4, 1980 issue of *Science News*, a small article reported that German researchers had had *smashing* success crushing kidney stones inside the body using shock waves generated outside the body. The technique, which eliminates the need for surgery, was conceived by Dornier System GmgH and developed in cooperation with both the Institution for Surgical Research and the Klinikum Grosshadern at Ludwig Maximilian University in Munich.

The article reported that clinical tests involving at least 16 patients were conducted earlier that year. Kidney stones were shattered into fragments so small that they were discharged naturally within a few days—"almost without discomfort."

Only three paragraphs were written in that 1980 publication regarding medical technology which has reformed today's treatment of kidney stones.

The Food and Drug Administration (FDA) approved the procedure for use in the United States in 1984.

> "..an authentic modern miracle."
>
> **Margaret Heckler on lithotripsy;**
> **former Secretary of Health and**
> **Human Services**

Today, when someone describes this procedure as completely safe, simple, easy or effortless, they are most likely comparing it to its alternative: conventional surgery, which carries a much higher risk of serious complications and requires a much longer hospital and recovery period.

My mother was thirty-five years old when she had kidney stone surgery. "One time was more than enough," my mother said remembering the pain of the surgery. "I stayed in the hospital nearly two weeks because I had three small children at home to care for," she said. "I needed the time to recover and the extra rest! It was extremely painful and something I never want to repeat again!"

In the thirty-seven years since her surgery, procedures for removing kidney stones have come a long way. Many advances have occurred in the last decade.

Just ask Jim Denman, a former newspaper photography editor. Thirteen years ago Denman underwent major surgery for the removal of a kidney stone. His eyes glaze over when he talks of it. After hearing of lithotripsy, he said, "I just can't believe how easy it is today compared to what I went through." The memory of his surgery, which left him recuperating at home for months, is a constant reminder to keep his fluid levels high so he can avoid repeat kidney stones. He now carries a gallon-sized jug of water on photo assignments—and has impressed other staff photographers to do the same.

Lithotripsy—How it Works

Lithotripsy, alone or in conjunction with other treatment, is an alternative to surgical removal for about 80 percent of those who suffer from kidney stones. The procedure utilizes an extracorporeal shock wave lithotripter (ESWL)—an out-of-body experience, you might say! The lithotripter is a machine which disintegrates kidney stones non-invasively.

Sounds like a monster from Mars? Neither the machine nor the procedure is to be feared!

The patient is positioned in a water tub or on a cushioned x-ray type of table, depending on which machine is used. An energy source produces shock waves outside the body which focus on the kidney stone within. These repeated shock waves cause the stone to crumble into tiny particles which are then passed out through the patient's urine. These shock waves pass through body tissue, causing no damage other than possible bruising.

Many individuals who have lithotripsy treatment experience little pain and can return to work within days. Compared to the severe pain and weeks of recovery after surgery, lithotripsy is "easy."

The Kidney Stone Center of Central California, which is operated by the Department of Urology at the University of California Davis Medical Center in Sacramento, has produced an excellent consumer information publication regarding lithotripsy. The brochure states that about two-thirds of those who could benefit from surgery can be effectively treated by lithotripsy alone. Of the remaining one-third, some will require additional procedures such as the placement of a catheter in the ureter or a tube through muscles of the back to help drain the kidney.

According to The Kidney Stone Center of Central California, about 20 percent of kidney stone sufferers have the type of stones which do not pass by themselves or have special conditions that require conventional surgery or other treatment. Special conditions that indicate other kinds of treatment include pregnancy, obesity (weight over 300 pounds) or extremes in height (shorter than four feet or taller than six feet, six inches). Patients with some types of cardiac pacemakers may not be able to undergo lithotripsy.

Persons with severe heart problems, bleeding disorders, physical malformations or other conditions may respond better to another kind of treatment. Additionally, to be eligible for lithotripsy, stones must be in the kidney or upper ureter and detectable by x-ray.

Most stones can be treated unless they're too small or irregularly shaped, or located in parts of the urinary system which are not in the kidney or upper ureter.

What to Expect Prior to Lithotripsy

Although details differ, a patient can expect the following general procedures:

- A few days before lithotripsy, the patient will receive a complete physical examination.
- X-rays, electrocardiogram, ultrasound, urinalysis, urine culture and blood tests may taken.
- Questions will be asked about the patient's medical history, including past operations, medications, allergies, etc.
- The patient may be asked to take a laxative or anti-gas product the evening before the scheduled lithotripsy.

While in the hospital or surgery center, a patient receives an IV (intravenous fluids) and is connected to monitors that check the pulse and blood pressure. Just prior to the procedure, some patients may be given a medication with a small sip of water which prevents nausea following surgery (useful if the patient has had anesthesia during the procedure).

To help an anxious patient relax during the treatment, the urologist may order a mild tranquilizer.

During Lithotripsy

The patient receives anesthesia—either general to allow the patient to sleep during treatment, or local, numbing the body from the waist down, or pain medication as needed. Although shock waves cause little harm to the patient, without some kind of anesthesia they may cause discomfort.

Another well-written brochure, from the Gallbladder and Kidney Stone Treatment Center at St. Mary Medical Center in Long Beach, California, describes how the procedure works. "During the procedure, the patient lies on an x-ray type table. The lithotripter uses x-ray and computer technology to pinpoint the shock wave at the stone's location. A water medium is necessary to transmit the shock wave to the stone. A water bag placed next to the patient's skin and a movable water column under the patient maintains a path between the patient and the shock wave generation point, permitting a dry environment" so that the patient is not immersed in a water bath as with other lithotripsy machines.

While there are several different types of extracorporeal shock wave lithotripsy (ESWL) units, the principles are the same for all. The stone is reduced into fine particles resembling sand.

Lithotripsy usually takes from 30 minutes to two hours to perform.

> It is important to inform the physician,
> anesthesiologist or nurse if any dis-
> comfort is felt. Ask all the questions
> you have.

Life After Lithotripsy

For a few days afterwards, the patient may experience some discomfort, fever, nausea or slight bleeding around the kidney (blood may be seen in the urine). These conditions, while not serious, can be treated with medication if necessary. It is suggested that the patient call his or her physician if such conditions occur.

The tiny stone particles will pass through the urine. Discomfort may be felt as these particles pass; it can be controlled with mild pain relievers.

The Northern California Kidney Stone Center recommends that following lithotripsy, patients perform a gravitation technique for lower pole stones. The Center feels this will improve passage of fragments through the urinary tract. The technique involves drinking water, then lying on an angled board, "head over head" twice a day following treatment.

It is suggested that patients use a rigid surface (such as an ironing board, exercise board or wooden planks) to form a 30 to 45 degree angled bed on which to lie during the process. The technique should begin one or two days following lithotripsy (or as soon as the patient feels recovered from the effects of anesthesia) and should be performed twice a day (morning and evening) for five to seven days following treatment.

The technique involves five steps. They include:

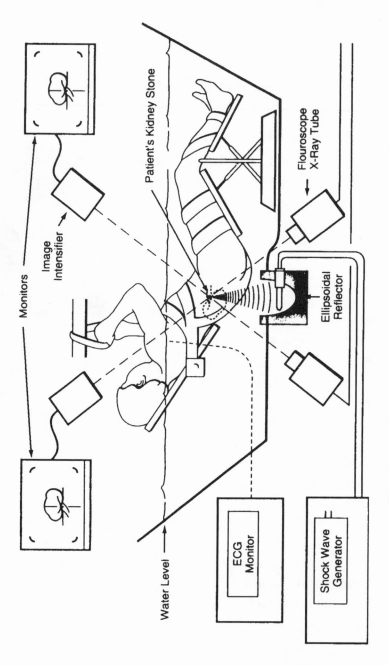

First-Generation Extracorporeal Shock Wave Lithotriptor
Illustration courtesy of Blaine Company Inc., Pharmaceuticals, Erlanger, Kentucky.

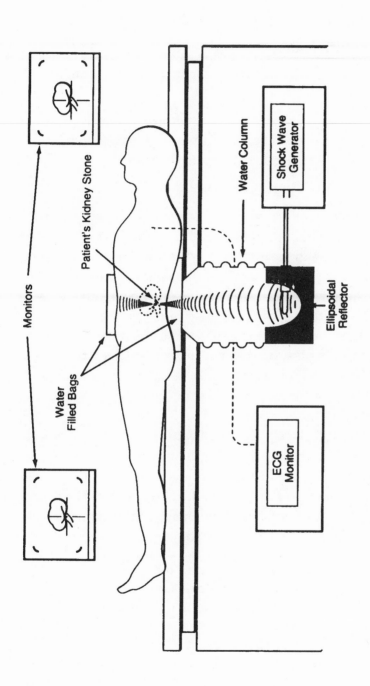

Second-Generation Extracorporeal Shock Wave Lithotriptor
Illustration courtesy of Blaine Company Inc., Pharmaceuticals, Erlanger, Kentucky.

1. Drink two 8-ounce glasses of water.

2. Wait 30 minutes.

3. Lie head down, face down for 30 minutes on your angled bed.

4. Lie on your side, head down, with your treated kidney up off the angled bed for 30 more minutes. If both kidneys were treated, alternate your position.

5. Get up and drink one 8-ounce glass of water.

The Kidney Stone Center also recommends jogging, running in place, jumping rope, or jumping jacks also to stimulate passage of stones in the ureters. Additionally, they suggest that during the first five to seven days following treatment, lie down or sleep with the treated kidney up. If both kidneys were treated, alternate the sleeping position periodically.

I tried the procedure and believe it helped. However, I found the ironing board extremely uncomfortable! Had I known about this procedure prior to lithotripsy, I would have obtained an exercise board to make the hour-long procedure far more comfortable.

In any event, even the ironing board was more comfortable than going through another urological treatment to remove stubborn kidney stone fragments!

The patient should continue to drink at least two quarts of water a day until all urinary symptoms have cleared up and all stone fragments have been passed.

Also important is using the urine strainer to recover stone fragments. Analyzing these fragments for their chemical content will help determine why they formed. With that information, the doctor can design a program to prevent recurrent episodes.

Most of my discomfort occurred when the stones were in my bladder. This, however, may not be true of most patients. Again, drinking large amounts of water helped to pass the stone fragments quickly. Also, I found it uncomfortable to sleep on the lithotripsy side. While the pain subsided after a few days, I was careful to keep from lying on that side. This eased the pain somewhat as well as encouraged stone passage.

If large or multiple stone fragments still remain, it is sometimes necessary to have additional lithotripsy or other treatments deemed necessary by your urologist.

Some patients will continue to pass stone fragments up to three months following lithotripsy—this is normal! One woman who wrote to me about her lithotripsy continued to stay in touch with weekly progress reports. She was very concerned that she had not passed any large stone fragments for almost six weeks following lithotripsy.

Finally, she decided to take a friend's large dog for a walk along the Pacific Grove coastline. "Well, actually the dog took me for a walk! It did the trick! When I got home, I passed two large stone fragments," she said.

I believe there is something to be said for remaining active following lithotripsy and letting gravity do its work!

Lithotripsy and the High Blood Pressure Question

In early 1990, it was reported in major United States newspapers that the use of shock waves to break up kidney stones appeared to increase blood pressure.

Doctors at Methodist Hospital of Indiana, located in Indianapolis, said patients showed a "small but significant" elevation in blood pressure two years after shock wave treatment.

They call the finding "cause for concern" even though the method of treatment still has overwhelming positive benefits.

Other published medical reports concluded that more studies are needed to determine what causes the blood pressure increases. *The British Journal of Urology* in 1991 reported that hypertension had been found in a small percentage of patients, again stressing that detailed studies are required. The researchers believe that lithotripsy is a safe procedure as far as renal function is concerned.

However, as recently as September 1992, Robert Gibbons, M.D., a urologist at Virginia Mason Medical Center in Seattle reported in a *Better Homes & Gardens* article that early reports linking lithotripsy to high blood pressure have been largely discounted.

Still, some physicians continue to advise their kidney stone patients to have their blood pressure checked at least two or three times a year thereafter as a precaution.

Survey results published for the urology profession in a medical journal reported most urologists questioned said they would prefer lithotripsy to surgery if they themselves had a renal stone that required removal.

What if I Have Only One Kidney?

Lithotripsy can be used as the treatment of first choice even when the kidney stone is in a single remaining kidney. *The Journal of Urology*, September 1992, reported a study from the Institute of Urology, University of Milan, Italy, in which Drs. Gianpaolo R. Zanetti, Emanuel Montanari and others found lithotripsy safe for patients who have a solitary kidney as a result of surgery. The researchers showed how the success rate—with the small number of complications at short-term follow-up, and the relatively small number of stone recurrences—proved lithotripsy a safe procedure.

The Cost for Lithotripsy

Lithotripsy is indeed safer and less painful, but not inexpensive. The charges for my second lithotripsy were $6,489.35 just for the procedure alone, with additional costs for both the anesthesiologist and the urologist.

One 5 mg. injection to keep me calm cost $32.00, and the *two* Alka Seltzer Gold given to settle my stomach were $8.00. If it would not put a protein load on my kidneys, I also expected to be given filet mignon at those prices!

I was fortunate to have insurance, although even with insurance coverage my out-of-pocket expenses left my budget financially drained. Perhaps money is another incentive as to why I feel I need to be as educated as possible to prevent any more stones. I'd rather spend my vacation dollars to a trip to the coast than on another kidney stone!

Looking to the Future

The long-term adverse effect of shock wave exposure remains to be established. Dr. James E. Lingeman of Methodist Hospital in Indianapolis wrote in an editorial in *The Journal of Urology* that properly designed clinical trials are still needed to examine these questions: What is the effect of lithotripsy on the growing kidneys of children? On blood pressure? What is the relationship of retained stone particles to risk of future new stone growth? Ultimately, Dr. Lingeman writes that appropriateness of any therapy rests upon balancing risk versus benefit. The long-term risks, (if any) associated with renal exposure to shock waves are yet to be adequately documented.

Lithotripsy is not likely to remain the "ultimate" in kidney stone treatment. Future innovations include a new device described as a "tiny jackhammer," which pulverizes kidney stones. The so-called "electromechanical impactor," developed by Massachusetts General Hospital (Boston) and Physical Sciences (an Andover, Massachusetts, research firm), uses a spring enclosed in a needle-like case that is inserted in the urinary track through a tube. Positioned near a stone, the metal head of the spring "hammers" against the stone until it breaks apart. The first human study results were presented at a bio-medical conference the first week in June 1991. The device proved successful for 14 of 16 patients with urinary tract stones.

According to a report in *Modern Healthcare* (June 10, 1991), it's hoped the device can be used with a local rather than general anesthetic.

The device is expected to be able to break up small kidney stones located in the ureters and on larger stones for which lithotripters haven't been as effective.

Other high-tech methods involve direct contact, threading something such as a laser into the urinary tract to break up the stone. These are invasive, require general or local anesthesia and carry the risk of complications such as scarring of the ureter. In the lower ureter, it's reasonable to use these tech-niques because the stone is near the outside of the body.

According to Dr. John A. Birkhoff's article in *Executive Health's Good Health Report* (June 1993) all contact techniques are done through a ureteroscope. This illuminated hollow metal tube can be passed up the urinary tract and into the bladder, where its special lenses, fiber optic lights and even cameras allow checks for inflam-mation, stones, or tumors.

Some techniques used in removing stones include electro-hydraulic lithotripsy, laser lithotripsy and ultrasonic lithotripsy.

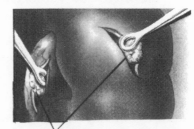

Surgical removal of stones from renal pelvis and kidney

Forceps   Basket   Electro-hydraulic   Laser

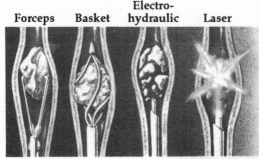

Extracorporeal shock wave lithotripsy

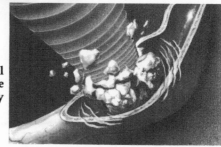

Illustrations courtesy of Blaine Company Inc., Pharmaceuticals, Erlanger, Kentucky.

Stone Free—Now What?

The procedure is over and finally, at long last—most patients are stone free! But not for long. Chances are greater than one in two that the patient will suffer another stone within five to seven years. Without preventative treatment, the average time between stone attacks is about a year and a half.

Following lithotripsy it's important to begin and continue preventative measures. Drinking large amounts of water, avoiding foods rich in the substances that made the stone, and perhaps taking a medication prescribed by the urologist can reduce the risk of future stones forming.

To find more information about lithotripsy, contact your physician, hospital or other health-care facility, kidney associations and local medical societies.

In the following section, you will read about my own experiences with lithotripsy. The professionals were right when they told me "don't worry!"

A Personal Story: Lithotripsy—
The Second Time Around

Three days after my second lithotripsy procedure, I went shopping at Macy's.

Perhaps the flashing neon lights, the new-clothes smell, and the ring of the cash register contributed to my overall good health. Within a few hours of the Macy's visit, I started to pass most of the larger stone fragments with only mild discomfort which was alleviated with pain medication.

Shopping does wonders for personal health!

Had you seen me a few days before the procedure, you would have seen a nervous and anxious patient—a true basket case. I like to joke that the "worry" gene is inherited from my father's side of the family.

During my "pre-op" visit with my urologist, I watched a video which explained what to expect during lithotripsy and what recovery would be like.

I related well to the patient in the video. She talked as she drove along the dramatic California coastline, famous for its wild hairpin turns. I have always loved the ocean. Yet, for the past three years, on every trip to the coast I brought not only an overnight bag, but also the fear that I might experience a kidney stone attack.

My greatest worry was being in a coastal community too small to have a hospital. In some places I have visited, the nearest facility was three hours away.

Concern was also expressed by the patient in the video. Imagine having freedom to travel anywhere without bringing along prescription pain medication, or having freedom to visit remote places that don't have a medical facility nearby. Imagine having one less huge piece of "baggage" on every trip.

My determination to be stone free helped me cope with my anxiety over what I thought was going to be yet another painful procedure.

Three years had elapsed since my first lithotripsy. New advancements in the type of lithotripter used, as well as new medical procedures, made lithotripsy more durable. I was amazed at the difference.

Three years previously, I required a "stent," a thin silastic tubing running from my kidney through my bladder to allow for safe passage of the shattered stone fragments, a spinal for anesthesia, a catheter, and a three-day hospitalization. While these medical procedures were not life threatening, they made life extremely uncomfortable, if not downright painful.

For the second lithotripsy, along with a rather large kidney stone, I brought on a lot of excess baggage from my first lithotripsy.

I expressed my concerns to my urologist and told him I was an anxious patient. He felt it best that I be given general anesthesia to make me "sleep." He explained how crucial it was that I not move during the procedure and that, if I did move, I could add 30 minutes to the procedure while the team searched for the exact location of the stone to resume the lithotripsy.

Additionally, the anesthesiologist explained during a "phone interview" the night before the procedure that anesthesia reduces respiratory movement and eliminates body movement.

I understood that quite well and liked the idea of sleeping through any and all discomfort. However, I wanted to remain awake since my goal was to write this section of the book which describes the procedure from my point of view. I couldn't do that asleep!

Following the visit with my urologist, I was given blood and urine tests at the out-patient surgery center. I completed a patient questionnaire for the staff anesthesiologist, filled out insurance forms, and signed hospital pre-admission forms in the unlikely event they were necessary. Then I was told to relax!

I remembered a story I was told years ago. Over the years it has most likely turned into a fractured fairy tale. In the story, Alice in Wonderland was crying. The Queen asked Alice why she was crying. "I am crying now so that when the time comes, I will not have anything to cry about," she said.

I view any procedure done to my own body this way. I do my crying before so I appear to be very brave when it actually happens.

The afternoon before the scheduled lithotripsy, I was given my own bottle of magnesium citrate which the drug company calls an "effervescent (fizzing) laxative." My doctor told me to drink the "pleasantly flavored laxative" at 4 p.m.

Luckily, the patient instructions warn that individual responses to laxatives vary and one should remain within easy access of toilet facilities. I never left home after 4 p.m. Needless to say, it worked.

> "Fortunately, kidney stones are seldom life-threatening, although they can temporarily take the joy out of existence."
>
> **—Allen J. Sheinman**
> **The Good News on Stones**
> **New Choices, August 1989**

I arrived at the surgery center at 8 a.m. the next day for a 10 a.m. lithotripsy. I had eaten nothing since midnight.

My doctor, however, had written an order for the surgical nurse to administer a mild tranquilizer, and since I wanted to continue feeling tranquil, I was glad to receive it.

I felt myself picking up on the fears of other patients who also waited to undergo surgical procedures at the out-patient surgery center. I felt their anxiety, tuned into it and listened to nurses' explanations. While I certainly empathized with both the nurses and patients, I needed to focus on remaining calm.

A friend stayed with me during that long two hour wait. Having someone to talk with helped me. The nurses were also helpful and answered all my questions...including some I didn't know to ask!

I also brought a tape player and some tranquil music which I eventually listened to rather than the conversations around me. Because music is soothing, I recommend that other patients undergoing lithotripsy check with their physicians about hospital policy regarding bringing in tapes and CD players.

The second-time-around lithotripsy did not require a catheter inserted into my bladder. I was delighted! Also, my urologist told me I most likely would not require a stent. Knowing that eased my fears.

Finally, it was my turn to travel on the gurney to the lithotripter. Two friendly nurses from the surgery center helped me "cruise" down the long surgery hallway on a gurney. The mobile kidney stone unit was "parked" behind the surgery center, and for a few seconds, I felt the warm summer sun on my face.

The gurney, with me on it, was placed on a lift. While it was no Disneyland thrill, I wondered how many patients were reminded of a carnival ride. That thought and the effects of the tranquilizer put a smile on my face. I idly wondered how many patients were dumped overboard when the lift malfunctioned.

At the touch of a button, I was lifted up to the mobile unit entrance (as if entering a warehouse). Once inside, however, I saw what looked like a friendly neighbor's living room nicely decorated with soothing wallpaper. I was amazed to find two artistic prints of the coast on the wall...I focused my thoughts on the places I loved.

During lithotripsy, the anesthesiologist plays an important role. He or she serves as a communicator between the patient, the lithotripsy staff and the physician. I found it extremely important to communicate my concerns and exactly how I was feeling to the anesthesiologist.

During my first lithotripsy, I did not communicate my fears or my pain to the anesthesiologist. I felt alone and unnecessarily uncomfortable as a result. As a quiet patient I endured more pain. During lithotripsy, it pays to be assertive!

When I voiced my opinion I was amazed by the positive changes. I received the high quality care I needed. I was a new lithotripsy patient the second time around—one who wasn't afraid to ask questions and knew what to expect!

Suddenly a new world of options opened as I moved onto the dry table of the lithotripter. I was again asked if I wanted general anesthesia or if I wanted to remain awake and receive pain medication as needed.

The anesthesiologist explained that if any part of the procedure was uncomfortable, I could safely be given anesthesia and, within a minute, be "put asleep." It was important that I remain awake to write this chapter, yet I thought preferable to be "asleep" because I was still anxious. Facing a last-minute decision, especially under the effects of a mild tranquilizer, left me uncertain.

I told the anesthesiologist I had no idea what I wanted; this proved the most frustrating part of the procedure.

With some of the newer machines, only a local anesthetic is needed. I was fortunate to have one of the newest units out on the market.

The staff suggested a decision regarding anesthesia: I would receive pain medication only as needed to see how well I could tolerate the procedure. The anesthesiologist conveyed my decision to the physician, who was surprised since I had spent considerable time explaining how anxious I was.

The procedure began.

X-ray devices within the lithotripter located the first of five stones in my right kidney within seconds. I felt the gentle nudging of the machine as it precisely positioned my right side. I had been told not to move—not even to scratch my nose! I was able to maintain that position during the entire one and a half hour-long procedure with minimal effort.

The greatest attention was given to two large kidney stones, one which was about the size of a quarter. Both were too large to pass through the ureter spontaneously.

With lithotripsy, neither soft tissues nor bones are hurt by the thousands of shock waves. The brittle stone, however, does absorb the shock waves and shatters under this impact, breaking into sand-like particles that are easier to pass in the urine.

I was able to use one of the newer, second-generation lithotripters that effectively uses low-power shock waves. With these machines, neither immersion in a water bath nor general anesthesia is usually necessary.

During the entire procedure, a loud noise directly above me resounded through the treatment room. As the procedure continued, the intensity of the shock waves could be felt—but was easily managed with pain medication. Two shock waves per second crumbled the stones.

During the treatment, x-rays determined the status of the stone. Typically, a stone begins to crumble after 200 to 400 shock waves.

I don't think ten minutes had passed before the lithotripsy technician who assisted my urologist walked over to me and held my hand. "Your stone has taken on a new form already, Gail," he said. "It's no longer in one piece."

As the procedure continued, I told the anesthesiologist when I needed more pain medication. Within seconds, the medication took effect and the pain was easily manageable. I was amazed how well it was going.

An hour and a half later, at the end of the procedure, I had received over 10,000 shock waves (similar to sound waves). Six thousand shock waves focused on one stone, and another 4,000 were sent into the smaller stone. Each shock wave carried a force of 5,000 to 15,000 pounds pressure per square inch. The force of a single shock wave, likened to a "hearty slap on the back," was more a "hearty slap in a very small area."

Finally, the room was silent.

It was over!

Once again I slid onto the gurney, and was wheeled out into the hot sun. My urologist, who walked next to my gurney, along with the two surgical nurses and the technician who had assisted, commented that lithotripsy patients should be given sunglasses as they're wheeled back to the surgery center.

But I was more than glad to see the sun! It was over!

Now it was important that I pass the stones by drinking large amounts of water. Following lithotripsy, my doctor advised me to drink lots of fluids to maintain a strong urinary flow and help eliminate the stone fragments. To recover those stone fragments, I filtered all my urine through the strainer the surgery center gave me.

Because I was not given general anesthesia, I was able to sit up in a lounge-type chair in the recovery room. However, I could not stop my body from shaking. The nurses theorized that my body was responding to the relief now that the procedure was over; the anesthesiologist feared that my blood sugar level was low since I had not eaten in over twelve hours.

Within minutes, I drank three small cans of apple juice and the shaking subsided.

I asked to use the bathroom, and though I was still connected to an IV unit, it felt wonderful to get up and walk. A recovery room nurse walked with me and stayed with me as I used the toilet. I was not prepared to see so much blood as I flushed the toilet. Before I could panic, the recovery room nurse told me bleeding was normal and it should subside within 24 to 48 hours.

In my case, it subsided in less than 24 hours—within 12 hours it appeared normal. Following lithotripsy, the patient should expect a pink or red discoloration of the urine for the first few days after treatment.

Also during the recovery room period, the nurse pointed out a red, four-inch round patch over my right kidney, a reaction to the lithotripsy. Some patients may find a small bruise. Although I was told to call my physician if the bruise got larger, it got smaller and disappeared by the fourth day.

The only discomfort I felt following the lithotripsy was a sore back over the right kidney which was easily managed with pain medication. I was too sore to sleep on my right side, but this too subsided within a week.

While it is not unusual to continue passing some stone fragments up to three months later, I passed the majority of the larger stone fragments by the fifth day. An x-ray examination two weeks after lithotripsy showed no stones. This was fantastic news!

Some patients experience pain, colic, fever or nausea during the first three months. These symptoms are of short duration and are treatable with mild pain medication.

Though lithotripsy is a relatively painless procedure, it is a physically taxing treatment. I was amazed how tired I was for a few days. A friend stayed with me and took over all household responsibilities—including cooking. This helped immensely. It also helped that my children spent some time with their dad. Several days of quiet, restful recovery without the responsibility of caring for others proved beneficial.

As I continued to pass the stone fragments, a friend asked me if I was "feeling like a beach?" He asked if I thought I should be at "Pebble Beach." Actually, I felt as if I were in a sand storm — but this was good news!

Overall, despite the discomfort, I have to say it didn't compare to my mother's long hospital stay, large scar from surgery and her long home recovery. Lithotripsy helped me get back to living life happily again without worrying about the pain of passing a kidney stone in the middle of the night...

...at some coastal hideaway in a remote area of Northern California.

Once again stone-free, I concentrated on better nutrition and eliminating the foods which could contribute to new kidney stones. Finding the information, however, was difficult. Then one day a nurse's book on nutrition for stone prone patients caught my eye in a medical library.

I had found gold! That information is now included in this book and the food charts can be found in the next chapter.

CHAPTER FIVE

Nutrition: What You Eat May Lead You Down the Rocky Road of Life

Benjamin Franklin is said to have stood on his head while eating blackberry jelly in an attempt to dislodge a stone in his bladder!

While he may been helping gravity dislodge stones by standing on his head, it's a different story for that blackberry jelly. The blackberry jelly, if his stone was made of calcium oxalate, may have contributed to further stone formation.

Today, with all the attention to high-tech treatments such as lithotripsy, we sometimes forget that patients with kidney stones can benefit from less glamorous therapies—like diet therapy.

Many experts believe that, while nutrition will not shock-wave stones into tiny pieces, it can help prevent their recurrence.

> "Food was becoming my 'enemy.' The foods I loved best seemed to be the ones contributing most to those painful stones."
>
> **—Gail Golomb**

Sweet potatoes and spinach, two of the few vegetables I really like, were now outlawed because of their oxalate content! Chocolate was high in oxalates? And to think I'd have to forego one of life's greatest pleasures! I drank gallons of iced tea in the summer, unaware that tea also contains substances which could form other stones in my kidneys.

Since foods may trigger the formation of kidney stones, doctors often recommend changing eating habits to prevent recurrences, whether or not drugs are prescribed.

An article in the *Canadian Medical Association* (January 1992) advises patients to seek individualized instruction from a qualified dietitian so diet is restricted as little as possible. The objective should be to limit excesses rather than curb intake completely.

Eating certain foods can increase mineral concentrations, yet few patients are given detailed lists of foods to avoid.

> Only 22 U.S. medical schools required a course on nutrition in 1989-1990. About 100 schools offered an elective course in nutrition, but only 5% of medical students took that elective according to a report in the *American Journal of Clinical Nutrition*.
>
> **University of California at Berkeley**
> ***Wellness Letter*, March 1992**
> **Published in association with**
> **The School of Public Health**

If such research is funded, future medical studies could shed new light on nutrition's important role in forming or preventing kidney stones.

Fish Oil for Sale!

One study focused on fish oil as a preventative for kidney stones. This study, reported in several United States newspapers during May, 1993 was conducted by Dr. A.C. Buck, a urologist with the Glasgow Royal Infirmary in Scotland. He presented his findings at the American Urological Association's annual meeting.

Fish oil was first examined by researchers after the discovery that Eskimos in Greenland lived on a diet of fatty fish, yet had low incidences of heart disease.

Dr. Buck reported that studies showed these Eskimos seldom had kidney stones. Certain oily fish such as mackerel, herring, sardines and salmon from cold northern seas appear to derive their benefits from a polyunsaturated fat known as omega-3 fatty acids.

In a three-month study of 40 patients suffering from recurrent kidney stones, the Glasgow researchers found that fish oil, alone or in combination with evening primrose oil, sharply reduced calcium levels in urine.

Dr. Buck believes that evening primrose oil, another polyunsaturated fatty acid, appears to boost the effects of fish oil.

Nutrients That Lead to Stone Formation

Nutrients which have been associated with calcium stone disease are dietary calcium, oxalate, protein, and sodium as well as alcohol and some fluids like tea or cola-flavored beverages.

Most studies, including one reported in *The Canadian Medical Association Journal* in January 1992, indicate that when stone-forming patients decrease calcium consumption, the result is decreased calcium excretion. However, these studies also indicate that decreasing calcium-containing foods without also decreasing oxalate (spinach, cocoa, tea, peanuts and rhubarb) also increases oxalate excretion. This carries an even greater risk for subsequent stone formation.

One of the newest nutrition studies, published in the *New England Journal of Medicine* (March 25, 1993), suggests that calcium-rich foods actually ward off rather than cause stones.

The Calcium Question

Physicians have encouraged kidney stone sufferers to steer clear of milk and other dairy foods to keep stones from returning. The recommendation seemed sensible since most kidney stones are largely calcium. Some urologists strongly believe that consuming dairy foods will put the stone patient back in their offices—again and again.

However, a new study from the Harvard School of Public Health found the opposite. Men who received lots of calcium in their diets (determined by responses to a food questionnaire) showed a one-third lower risk of stone formation than the patients who consumed little calcium.

Harvard researcher Dr. Gary C. Curhan warned patients that "the important message is that people who have had calcium stones should not restrict their calcium intake. People may actually be at increased risk of forming stones if they do."

While the study was conducted entirely on men—45,619 of them—Dr. Curhan believes the findings will also apply to women. Good news, since women have even more reason to consume lots of calcium which reduces their higher risk of bone fractures due to osteoporosis.

At the start of the 1986 study, none of the men had ever had kidney stones. In the four years of follow-up studies, 505 participants who had never had previous stones, developed them.

Among the results published in the *New England Journal of Medicine:*

- The quarter of men with the highest calcium consumption had a 34 percent lower risk of stones than did the quarter with the lowest intake.

- Men with the highest consumption of potassium, which is contained in fruits and vegetables, had only half the risk of developing kidney stones.

- A high fluid intake was associated with a 29 percent lower risk.

In an accompanying editorial, Dr. Jacob Lemann, Jr. of the Medical College of Wisconsin called the study impressive. In view of this report, he wrote that, for stone sufferers, "there is no benefit to the time-honored advice to eat a diet low in calcium."

Why calcium might be good rather than bad is unclear. However, Harvard researchers speculated the answer might relate to another component of kidney stones: oxalate.

Foods high in oxalate may increase the risk of stones, and calcium may block its absorption in the kidneys.

Curhan recommended that people worried about stones make sure they get the recommended daily allowance of calcium (about 800 milligrams for most adults). This is the equivalent of just over three 8-ounce glasses of milk. The recommended amount for pregnant and nursing women is 1,200 milligrams.

Dietary intake of animal fat was directly associated with risk of stone formation while a diet high in fluids and potassium-containing foods decreased the risk of kidney stones.

Since it's not unprecedented for conventional wisdom to turn out wrong, the wise patient should continue to consult with their physician concerning dietary calcium, as well as calcium supplements.

Other researchers do not recommend that people who have already had a stone or who have a family history of kidney stones should increase their calcium intake on the basis of this single study, which they feel raises more questions than it answers. The study looked at men who initially never had stones. The finding may or may not apply to men with a previous history of stones, or to women. And there may have been something else, still unidentified, in the diet or lifestyle of the men in the study who consumed lots of calcium.

The Calcium Information Center (1-800-321-2681) advises patients with kidney stones to contact their health care provider before beginning supplemental calcium.

Some studies suggest that if calcium is severely restricted (to less than 400 mg. a day), this may result in osteoporosis over a long period of time. The physician's dietary prescription will have to take into account the patient's age and sex.

Because most patients with calcium stones excrete too much calcium in their urine, many physicians order thiazide diuretics to reduce calcium. Cutting back on table salt and high-sodium foods may also help. Since sodium and calcium compete for reabsorption in the kidney, the less sodium that reaches the renal tube, the more calcium will be reabsorbed into the blood. This event will keep urinary calcium low.

A high-protein diet also leads to increased calcium in the urine. These diets tend to lower the urinary pH and can increase uric acid. Additionally, a low pH may also reduce kidney stone inhibitors by decreasing citrate in the urine.

New York Hospital-Cornell Medical Center and **Oregon Health Sciences University** operate a toll-free telephone number that provides recorded information about calcium intake. The number is (800) 321-2681. Leave your name, address, phone number and question. You can expect a response back in about a week.

Or write to:

The Calcium Information Center, *New York Hospital-Cornell Medical Center, 515 East 71st St., S-904, New York, NY 10021.*

They offer a free, excellent publication on "Calcium Close-Ups: Every Woman's Guide to a Vital Nutrient."

The National Center for Nutrition and Dietetics *can provide answers to diet and nutritional questions by mail or telephone. Call: (312) 899-4853.*

Or write to:

National Center for Nutrition and Dietetics, *American Dietetic Association, 216 West Jackson Blvd., Suite 800, Chicago, IL 60606-6995*

Since people with stones tend to excrete high levels of oxalate in their urine, stone formers may be eating more oxalate-rich foods. For example, spinach has 1,350 mg. of oxalate per serving; rhubarb 1,092 mg. and baked beans 50 mg. Swiss chard and beet greens each contain 1,000 mg.

According to a medical progress report published in *The New England Journal of Medicine*, October 15, 1992 by Fredric L. Coe, M.D., Joan H. Parks, M.B.A., and John R. Asplin, M.D., a simple dietary excess of oxalate increases urinary oxalate up to 50 to 60 mg daily. Specifically, foods such as spinach, rhubarb, Swiss chard, cocoa, beets, peppers, wheat germ, pecans, peanuts, okra, chocolate and lime peel are all suspect.

Treatment for patients with hyperoxaluria includes altering the diet to avoid excess oxalate. Patients should make follow-up visits so their physicians can test their urine and blood.

The Case for Less Animal Protein

As stated previously, a diet high in animal protein is linked with stone formation. This may be why the number of Americans who are stone prone is increasing.

We seem to have a mismatch between the evolutionary design of our kidneys and the functional burden we place on them by our modern eating habits. The average meat-eating American consumes 100 grams of protein per day, two to three times the Recommended Dietary Allowance, with most of the protein coming from animal products.

According to the January 1992 issue of *Vegetarian Times*, research indicates that vegetarians, providing they do not overdose on dairy products and eggs, are less likely to encounter kidney stones "on the rocky road of life."

Researchers from University Hospital in Leiden, Netherlands, conducted a study to find out why too much protein could lead to kidney stones. They put healthy men on two levels of protein, an average base level of 80 grams per day and a high level of 160 grams.

Study results showed that the men on the higher protein diet experienced significant chemical changes in their urine, increasing the likelihood of kidney-stone formation. The men also consumed varying levels of sodium, and similar changes took place. When high animal-protein and high sodium diets were combined, even more significant chemical changes occurred.

Because the study looked at only one small group of patients, researcher Dik J. Kok, M.D., isn't ready to recommend less protein—yet.

Since people react differently, limiting animal protein intake may become the dietary regimen of choice.

Again, patients will need to consult their physicians or a dietician if substituting a meat-rich diet for a vegetarian diet due to oxalates found in many vegetables. Food charts at the end of this chapter will be helpful to patients wishing to avoid foods high in oxalate.

Uric Acid Stones and Diet

Uric acid is also affected by diet. Patients with a diet rich in animal protein almost double the uric acid in their urine. Uric acid is a product of purine, which is found primarily in animal protein.

Unlike calcium oxalate stones, uric acid stones dissolve once urinary pH rises (unless they are coated with calcium oxalate). Physicians often prescribe Allopurinol (Zyloprim) to reduce the uric acid level in the urine of patients with uric acid stones. A patient with gout who develops stones while taking Probenecid (Benemid)—which increases urinary uric acid levels—may be switched to another drug, such as Colchinine.

The role alcoholic beverages play in diet can be significant. Both wine and spirits can impair the ability of kidneys to eliminate uric acid from the blood. Thus, patients who have restricted their diet due to uric acid must be prudent with their use of alcohol; some are advised to eliminate it entirely, at least until appropriate urate-lowering drugs have had a chance to work.

> The richest food sources of uric acid are anchovies, asparagus, liver, kidney, sardines, meat extracts, and mushrooms.

Kidney Stones: The Disease of Affluence

The June, 1991 issue of *Nutrition Research Newsletter* reports that diet is believed to be a major contributor to the high rate of kidney stones in affluent countries. The article reported the findings of Dr. A. Trinchieri and others on "The Influence of Diet on Urinary Risk Facts for Stones in Healthy Subjects."

The authors believe that "renal stone formers could be predisposed to stones because of their dietary patterns." The findings suggest that a 'rich' diet makes men more prone to calcium stones than women, whereas metabolic abnormalities play a prominent part in stone formation in women.

The researchers also note that these and previous findings may differ due to sample and control groups used.

A Japanese study reported in the *Nutrition Research Newsletter*, November 1990, that kidney stone disease in Japan has tripled since World War II, a change linked to the westernization of the Japanese diet. In a previous study, researchers from Kinki University in Osaka found that men with kidney stone disease ate more protein and less calcium than did healthy men, and often ate large, late dinners with short intervals between dinner and retiring.

The authors believe that "individual dietary management should be the primary measure" for preventing kidney stone disease in Japan.

Still more medical research points a finger at food as the leading cause of kidney stones. *The Journal of the Canadian Dietetic Association* reported in Fall, 1990 that patients who significantly decreased their protein, calcium and oxalate intakes and increased their water intake while on this modified diet were less likely to form stones.

Kidney Stones and Dietary Fiber

In the study above, which was conducted at Halifax (Nova Scotia) Infirmary Hospital, patients were given dietary fiber consisting of two high-fiber biscuits (wheat-bran or corn-bran biscuits). Placed on a modified diet with increased fluids, limited calcium (500-700 mg/day), no more than 40-60 mg/day of oxalate, and 35-55 g/day of animal protein for three months, including two high-fiber biscuits for four weeks, the patients showed fiber decreased the urinary calcium and oxalate levels.

Rice Bran and Vitamins

In another published medical report in the *Nutrition Research Newsletter* (June 1991), researchers found that defatted rice bran (which contains phytin) binds calcium in the intestine and decreases urinary calcium output. This may prevent calcium stones from recurring in hypercalciuric patients.

The study followed 49 patients who received rice bran for more than three years. The results showed an obvious decline in stone formation rate, as compared with the three years immediately preceding treatment. In 30 patients (61.2 percent), no new stones formed during rice bran treatment.

The authors suggest that, while rice bran therapy is effective in reducing the recurrence of calcium stones in hypercalciuric patients, combining it with other preventative measures may be necessary for its effectiveness.

Vitamin B6 and Magnesium

In an article appearing in *Prevention Magazine* (September 1989), Kerry Pechter reports on the advice Alan Wasserstein, M.D., director of the Stone Evaluation Center at the Hospital of the University of Pennsylvania gives his patients. As additional insurance, Dr. Wasserstein often prescribes vitamin B6 and magnesium supplements because he feels they tend to reduce oxalate levels and inhibit stone formation in some people.

Other reports also suggest that vitamin B6 and magnesium supplements help. Magnesium is less likely than calcium to form kidney stones when it binds with oxalate in urine. Since magnesium and calcium compete for oxalate, the chances of calcium coming out as the "winner" are reduced—as are the chances of getting stones.

> *The Inside Story: What You Need to Know About Your Digestive System*, from the editors of Rodale Press, includes a report by researchers in Boston on a long-term study of 149 patients. Results showed a 90 percent cut in calcium oxalate stone formation after daily nutritional therapy. The nutrients: magnesium and vitamin B6.

Canadian researchers report similar results with these vitamin supplements. An article in the *Canadian Health Foods Association Newsletter* (October 1990), suggested that supplementing the diet with vitamin B6 and magnesium helps reduce oxalate levels and keeps kidney stones from forming.

Drugs which reduce magnesium levels include digitalis and oral diuretics.

Good food sources of magnesium include leafy, green vegetables (eaten raw), nuts (especially almonds and cashews), soybeans, seeds and whole grains.

On April 6, 1992, a *TIME* magazine cover story reported that vitamins promise to unfold as one of the great and hopeful health stories of our day.

TIME reported that the National Institutes of Health, universities, and other research organizations have begun funding laboratory and clinical investigations. By the late 1980's, research exploring vitamins' potential in protecting against disease was on its way to respectability. "Though the evidence is still preliminary, scientists are excited about several nutrients," the article stated.

The Nutrition Desk Reference by Robert H. Garrison, Jr., M.A., and Elizabeth Somer, M.D., suggests that kidney stones may be a deficiency of vitamin B6. Overall, evidence is strong that vitamin B6 and magnesium is significant in kidney stone prevention.

> "As I see it, except for these supplements (250 to 500 milligrams of magnesium and 10 to 20 milligrams of vitamin B6), nothing more is needed either to prevent or dissolve kidney or bladder stones than a diet that furnishes adequate amounts of every nutrient including calcium."
>
> **Adelle Davis**
> *Let's Get Well*

Kidney Stones Vs. Osteoporosis:
To Be Or Not To Be

The fear of osteoporosis surfaces when stone diets restrict calcium intake. For women, this is a serious concern.

One benefit of Vitamin D (produced when the skin is exposed to sunlight) is that it may prevent osteoporosis. For women who have been told to restrict their calcium consumption due to kidney stones, yet worry about developing osteoporosis, this is indeed welcome news.

After asking about limiting my calcium and thus increasing my chance of developing osteoporosis later in life, I was advised outdoor activity and exercise would lessen my risk of osteoporosis.

During the summer of 1992, newspapers reported that Indianapolis researchers believed they found the reason post-menopausal women often have the weak-bone condition called osteoporosis. Dr. Stavros C. Manolagas of the Veterans Medical Center and Indiana University School of Medicine in Indianapolis said laboratory studies show that a lack of the hormone estrogen leads to overproduction of bone scavenger cells that carve pits and craters throughout the skeleton.

The finding may lead to new drugs or therapies to combat the disorder.

For those in danger of osteoporosis who don't want to restrict calcium intake, some physicians suggest one way to keep calcium in the bones and out of the bloodstream is to take Diural or another of the thiazides, a group of diuretics.

Another option is oral phosphates which tend to bind calcium in the intestines so less is absorbed.

However, dietary changes show the same improvement in stone recurrence as thiazides. Medication should be reserved for people who keep making stones despite changes in their diet, or who can not manage to change their diets or drinking habits.

Some patients, even those on a low-calcium diet, for unknown reasons may excrete as much as 500 mg. of calcium daily.

Diet and Kidney Stones

Are all kidney stones the same?

No. Kidney stones are made of different substances and have different causes. The treatment for kidney stones is not the same for everyone.

Is there a diet I can follow to prevent stones? How will I know what diet changes are right for me?

You may need to follow a special diet. First your doctor will need to run tests to find out why you form stones and what diet changes may be right for you. You may be asked to use less salt, calcium, oxalate, or animal protein in your diet. Your registered dietitian will be able to plan your diet.

Will following a special diet mean I will not have to take my medicines?

Sometimes, following a special diet may be enough to prevent you from forming more kidney stones. Other times, medicines may also need to be taken.

I had a calcium stone. Should I avoid calcium?

Not necessarily. You might put out large amounts of calcium in your urine even if you do not eat high calcium foods. There are special tests that can find out if you need to limit the amount of calcium you eat. However, if you eat large amounts of high calcium foods, it would be a good idea to cut back some until you can be tested.

What foods are good sources of calcium?

Dairy products such as milk, cheese, ice cream, and yogurt are high in calcium. Other high calcium foods are sardines or salmon canned with bones, oysters and tofu. Some foods have extra calcium added (for example, some cold cereals and instant oatmeal), and some medicines have large amounts of calcium.

I am worried about developing osteoporosis if I limit the calcium in my diet. How can I protect my bones from becoming weak and brittle as I get older?

You need about 800 to 1000 milligrams of calcium per day. If you eat a diet with less calcium over a long period of time you may have a loss of bone. Most people get about two thirds of their calcium from dairy products. A dietitian can help you to choose the right food to get enough calcium to meet your needs.

My kidney stone contained oxalate. Do I need to avoid all foods high in oxalate?

Sometimes eating foods with a lot of oxalate can make conditions right for you to form a stone. In this case, limiting foods high in oxalate may be helpful. However, avoiding foods high in oxalate is not necessary for all people who form stones.

What are some of the foods high in oxalate?

Foods with a high content of oxalate include peanuts, peanut butter, tea, rhubarb, beets, spinach and other dark, leafy greens, sweet potato, chocolate, and tofu.

I have had calcium oxalate stones in the past. My doctor tells me to avoid salt. What does salt have to do with calcium oxalate?

A high salt intake can increase the amount of calcium in your urine. Extra calcium in the urine can cause you to form stones. Also, if you are being treated with a thiazide medicine as part of your treatment and you have a high salt intake, the medicine may be less effective.

My doctor told me to drink a lot of fluids. How much is "a lot?" Why is this important?

You should drink at least 12 to 16 cups (3 to 4 quarts or liters) of fluid throughout the day. Most of this should be water. Drinking this amount will allow your kidneys to make at least 2 1/2 quarts of urine—the amount necessary to prevent new kidney stones. In hot weather you should drink more fluids (above 4 quarts) to make up for fluid lost as sweat. Drinking more fluids should dilute the chemical salts in your urine and prevent their forming a stone. Do not drink bottled or mineral water until you get more information from a dietitian. If you live in a hard water area, mention this to the dietitian.

Will it help/hurt me to take a vitamin or mineral supplement?

The B vitamins (which include thiamine, riboflavin, niacin, B6 and B12) have not been shown to be harmful to people with kidney disease. However, taking vitamin C, vitamin D, fish liver oil, or mineral supplements containing calcium can increase the chances of stone formation in some people. You should take vitamin and/or mineral supplements ONLY on the advice of your doctor or dietitian.

Reprinted from The National Kidney Foundation, Inc. Developed by The National Kidney Foundation Council on Renal Nutrition; 1991 04-06NN, Kidney and Urology Facts.

Today the good news is that one does not have to return to the Stone Age to prevent kidney stones from occurring. Most physicians simply advise their patients to go back to basics—fresh fruits and vegetables, nuts, seeds and whole-grain products, less meat and less fat.

The food charts on the following pages will help you avoid the foods rich in the substances which formed your kidney stone.

Nutrition Charts

Food Sources of Oxalates:
Calcium-Oxalate Stones

Fruits	Vegetables	Nuts	Beverages	Other
Berries, all	Baked beans	Almonds	Chocolate	Grits
Currants	Beans, green	Cashews	Cocoa	Tofu, soy
Concord	and wax	Peanuts	Draft beer	products
grapes	Beets	Peanut butter	Tea	Wheat germ
Figs	Beet greens			
Fruit cocktail	Celery			
Plums	Chard, Swiss			
Rhubarb	Chives			
Tangerines	Collards			
	Eggplant			
	Endive			
	Kale			
	Leeks			
	Mustard greens			
	Okra			
	Peppers, green			
	Rutabagas			
	Spinach			
	Squash, summer			
	Sweet potatoes			
	Tomatoes			
	Tomato soup			
	Vegetable soup			

Low-Calcium Diet: Calcium Stones
(approximately 400 mg calcium)

	Foods Allowed	Foods Not Allowed
Beverage	Carbonated beverage, coffee, tea	Chocolate-flavored milk, milk drinks
Bread	White and light rye bread or crackers	
Cereals	Refined cereals	Oatmeal, whole-grain cereals
Desserts	Cake, cookies, gelatin desserts, pastries, pudding, sherbets, all made without chocolate; milk or nuts. If egg yolk is used, it must be from one egg allowance.	
Fat	Butter, cream, 2 tbsp daily; French dressing, margarine, salad oil, shortening	Cream (except in amount allowed), mayonnaise
Fruits	Canned, cooked, or fresh fruits or juice except rhubarb	Dried fruit, rhubarb
Meats, eggs	8 oz. daily of any meat, fowl, or fish except clams, oysters, or shrimp; not more than one egg daily including those used in cooking.	Clams, oysters, shrimp, cheese
Potato or substitute	Potato, hominy, macaroni, noodles, refined rice, spaghetti	Whole-grain rice
Soup	Broth, vegetable soup made from vegetables allowed	Bean or pea soup, cream or milk soup
Sweets	Honey, jam, jelly, sugar	
Vegetables	Any canned, cooked, or fresh vegetables or juice except those listed	Dried beans, broccoli, green cabbage, celery, chard, collards, endive, greens, lettuce, lentils, okra, parsley, parsnips, dried peas, rutabagas
Misc.	Herbs, pickles, popcorn, relishes, salt, spices, vinegar	Chocolate, cocoa, milk gravy, nuts, olives, white sauce

Note: Depending on calcium content of local water supply, in instances of high calcium content, distilled water may be indicated.

Low-Calcium Test Diet
(200 mg calcium)

	Grams	Milligrams Calcium
Breakfast		
Orange Juice, fresh	100	19.00
Bread (toast), white	25	19.57
Butter	15	3.00
Rice Krispies	15	3.70
Cream, 20% butterfat	35	33.95
Sugar	7	0.00
Jam	20	2.00
Distilled water, coffee, or tea*		0.00
TOTAL		**81.22**
Lunch		
Beef steak, cooked	100	10.00
Potato	100	11.00
Tomatoes	100	11.00
Bread	25	19.57
Butter	15	3.00
Honey	20	1.00
Applesauce	20	1.00
Distilled water, coffee or tea		0.00
TOTAL		**56.57**
Dinner		
Lamb chop, cooked	90	10.00
Potato	100	11.00
Frozen green peas	80	10.32
Bread	25	19.57
Butter	15	3.00
Jam	20	2.00
Peach sauce	100	5.00
Distilled water, coffee or tea		0.00
TOTAL		**60.89**
TOTAL MILLIGRAMS CALCIUM		**198.68**

use distilled water only for cooking and beverages

Low-Phosphorus Diet: Struvite Stones
(approximately 1 g phosphorus and 40 g protein)

(Struvite stones are composed of a simple compound, magnesium ammonium phosphate ($MgNH_4PO_4$). These are often called infection stones because they are associated with urinary tract infections.)

	Foods Allowed	Foods Not Allowed
Milk	Not more than 1 cup daily; whole, skim or buttermilk or 3 tbsp. powered, including the amount used in cooking	Milk and milk drinks except as allowed
Beverages	Fruit juices, tea, coffee, carbonated drinks, Postum	
Bread	White only; enriched commercial, French, hard rolls, soda crackers, rusk	Rye and whole-grain breads, cornbread, biscuits, muffins, waffles
Cereals	Refined cereals, such as Cream of Wheat, Cream of Rice, rice, cornmeal, dry cereals, cornflakes, spaghetti, noodles	All whole-grain cereals
Desserts	Berry or fruit pies, cookies, cakes in average amounts; Jell-O, gelatin, angel food cake, sherbet, meringues made with egg whites, pudding if made with one egg or milk allowance.	Desserts with milk and eggs, unless made with the daily allowance
Eggs	Not more than one egg daily, including those used in cooking; extra egg whites may be used	
Fats	Butter, margarine, oils, shortening	
Fruits	Fresh, frozen, canned, as desired	Dried fruits such as raisins, prunes, dates, figs, apricots

Low-Phosphorus Diet: Struvite Stones
(continued)

	Foods Allowed	Foods Not Allowed
Meat	One large serving or two small servings daily of beef, lamb, veal, pork, rabbit, chicken or turkey	Fish, shellfish (crab, oyster, shrimp, lobster, and so on), dried and cured meats (bacon, ham, chipped beef, and so on), liver, kidney, sweetbreads, brains
Cheese	None	Avoid all cheese and cheese spreads
Vegetables	Potatoes as desired; at least two servings per day of any of the following: asparagus, carrots, beets, green beans, squash, lettuce, rutabagas, tomatoes, celery, peas, onions, cucumber, corn; no more than 1 serving daily of either cabbage, spinach, broccoli, cauliflower, brussel sprouts, or artichokes	Dried vegetables such as peas, mushrooms, lima beans
Misc.	Sugar, jams, jellies, syrups, salt, spices, seasonings; condiments in moderation	

Sample Menu

Breakfast	Lunch	Dinner
Fruit juice	Meat (2 oz.)	Meat (2 oz)
Refined cereal	Potato	Potato
Egg	Vegetable	Vegetable
White toast	Salad	Salad
Butter	Bread, white	Bread, white
1/2 cup milk	Butter	Butter
Coffee or tea	1/2 cup milk	Dessert
	Dessert	Coffee or tea
	Coffee or tea	

Acid Ash Diet: Calcium Stones

The purpose of this diet is to furnish a well-balanced diet in which the total acid ash is greater than the total alkaline ash each day. It lists (1) unrestricted foods, (2) restricted foods, (3) food not allowed, and (4) sample of a day's diet.

Unrestricted Foods
Eat as much as desired of the following foods

Bread	any, preferably whole grain, crackers, rolls
Cereals	any, preferably whole grain
Desserts	angel food or sunshine cake, cookies made without baking powder or soda; cornstarch pudding, cranberry desserts, custards, gelatin desserts, ice cream, sherbet, plum or prune desserts, rice or tapioca pudding
Fats	any, as butter, margarine, salad dressings, shortening, lard, salad oils, olive oil
Fruits	cranberries, plums, prunes
Meat, eggs, cheese	any meat, fish, or fowl, two servings daily; at least one egg daily
Potato substitutes	corn, hominy, lentils, macaroni, noodles, rice, spaghetti, vermicelli
Soup	broth as desired, other soups from foods allowed
Sweets	cranberry or plum jelly; sugar, plain sugar candy
Misc.	cream sauce, gravy, peanut butter, peanuts, popcorn, salt, spices, vinegar, walnuts

Restricted Foods
Do not eat any more than the amount allowed each day.

Milk   2 cups daily (may be used in other ways than as beverage)
Cream: 1/3 cup or less daily

Fruits   one serving of fruit daily (in addition to prunes, plums, cranberries)

Vegetables including potato   two servings daily; certain vegetables listed under "Foods not allowed" are not allowed at any time.

Foods Not Allowed

carbonated beverages, such as ginger ale, cola, root beer

cakes or cookies made with baking powder or soda

Fruits   dried apricots, bananas, dates, figs, raisins, rhubarb

Vegetables   dried beans, beet greens, dandelion greens, carrots, chard, lima beans

Sweets   chocolate or candies other than those under "unrestricted foods;" syrups

Miscellaneous   other than peanuts and walnuts, nuts, olives, pickles

---

Sample Menu

Breakfast	**Lunch**	**Dinner**
Grapefruit	Creamed chicken	Broth
Wheatena	Steamed rice	Roast beef, gravy
Scrambled eggs	Green beans	Buttered noodles
Toast, butter, plum jam	Stewed prunes	Sliced tomato
Coffee, cream, sugar	Bread, butter	Mayonnaise
	Milk	Bread, butter
		Vanilla ice cream

Low-Purine Foods: Uric Acid Stones

Foods from this list may be used as desired; these foods contain an insignificant amount of purine.

Beverages
  Carbonated
  Chocolate
  Cocoa
  Coffee
  Fruit juices
  Postum
  Tea
Butter*
Bread
  white and crackers
  cornbread
Cereals and cereal products
  Corn
  Rice
  Tapioca
  Refined wheat
  Macaroni
  Noodles
Cheese of all kinds*

Eggs
Fats of all kinds*
  (moderation)
Fruits of all kinds
Gelatin, Jell-O®
Milk
  buttermilk,
  evaporated, malted,
  sweet
Nuts of all kinds*,
  peanut butter*
Pies*
  (except mincemeat)
Sugar and sweets
Vegetables
  Artichokes
  Beets
  Beet greens
  Broccoli
  Brussels sprouts
  Cabbage

Carrots
Celery
Corn
Cucumber
Eggplant
Endive
Kohlrabi
Lettuce
Okra
Parsnips
Potato, white and
  sweet
Pumpkin
Rutabagas
Sauerkraut
String beans
Summer squash
Swiss chard
Tomato
Turnips

high in fat

The foods in the following list contain a moderate amount (up to 75 mg) of purine in 200 g serving. Serve one item four times a week.

Asparagus
Bluefish
Bouillon
Cauliflower
Chicken
Crab
Finnan haddie
Ham

Herring
Kidney beans
Lima beans
Lobster
Mushrooms
Mutton
Navy beans
Oatmeal

Oysters
Peas
Salmon
Shad
Spinach
Tripe
Tuna fish
Whitefish

The following list contains foods that contain a large amount (75-150 mg) of purine in 100 g. serving; one item once a week.

Bacon	Lentils	Quail
Beef	Liver sausage	Rabbit
Calf tongue	Meat soups	Sheep
Carp	Partridge	Shellfish
Chicken Soup	Perch	Squab
Codfish	Pheasant	Trout
Duck	Pigeon	Turkey
Goose	Pike	Veal
Halibut	Pork	Venison

Avoid entirely; foods that contain very large amounts (150-1000 mg) of purine in 100 g serving.

Sweetbreads	825 mg.	Kidneys (beef)	200 mg
Anchovies	363 mg.	Brains	195 mg.
Sardines (in oil)	295 mg.	Meat extracts	(160-400 mg)
Liver (calf, beef)	233 mg.	Gravies	Variable

Typical Meal Pattern

Breakfast	**Lunch**	**Dinner**
Fruit	Egg or cheese dish	Egg or cheese dish
Refined cereal and/or egg	Vegetables, as allowed (cooked or salad)	Cream of vegetable soup, if desired
White toast	Potato or substitute	Starch (potato or substitute)
Butter, 1 tsp	White bread	Colored vegetable, as allowed
Sugar	Butter, 1 tsp	White bread
Coffee	Fruit or simple dessert	Butter, 1 tsp if desired
Milk, if desired	Milk	Salad, as allowed
		Fruit or simple dessert
		Milk

Low-Methionine Diet: Cystine Stones

	Foods Allowed	Foods Not Allowed
Soup	Any soup made without meat stock or addition of milk	Rich meat soups, broths, canned soups made with meat broth
Meat or meat substitute	Peanut butter sandwich, spaghetti, or macaroni dish made without addition of meat, cheese, or milk; one serving day day: chicken, lamb, veal, beef, pork, crab, or bacon (3)	Fish and those not listed above
Beverages	Soy milk, tea, coffee	Milk in any form
Vegetables	Asparagus, artichoke, beans, beets, carrots, chicory, cucumber, eggplant, escarole, lettuce, onions, parsnips, potatoes, pumpkin, rhubarb, tomatoes, turnips	Those not listed as allowed
Fruits	Apples, apricots, bananas, berries, cherries, fruit cocktail, grapefruit, grapes, lemon juice, nectarines, oranges, peaches, pears, pineapple, plums, tangerines, watermelon, cantaloupe	Those not listed as allowed
Salads	Raw or cooked vegetable or fruit salad	
Cereals	Macaroni, spaghetti, noodles	
Bread	Whole wheat, rye, white	
Nuts	Peanuts	
Desserts	Fresh or cooked fruit, ices, fruit pies	
Eggs		In any form
Cheese		All varieties
Concentrated sweets	Sugar, jams, jellies, syrup, honey, hard candy	
Concentrated fats	Butter, margarine, cream	
Misc.	Pepper, mustard, vinegar, garlic, oil, herbs, spices	

Meal Pattern

Breakfast	Lunch	Dinner
1 cup fruit juice	1 serving soup	2 oz. meat
1/2 cup fruit	1 serving sandwich	1 med. starch
1 slice toast	1 cup fruit	1/2 cup vegetable
1 1/2 pats butter	8 oz. soy milk*	1 serving salad
2 tsp jelly	3 tsp sugar	1 tbsp dressing
1 tbsp sugar	1 tbsp cream	1 slice bread
Beverage	Beverage	1 serving dessert
1 tbsp cream		1 tbsp cream
		1 1/2 pats butter
		Beverage

Optional: use for children to include protein intake.
Omit if urine calcium is elevated in adults.

Sample Menu

Breakfast	Lunch	Dinner
Orange juice	Vegetable soup,	Chicken, roast
Applesauce	vegetarian	Baked potato
Whole-wheat toast	Peanut butter sandwich	Artichoke
Butter	Canned peaches	Sliced tomatoes
Jelly	Soy milk*	French dressing
Sugar	Sugar	Whole-wheat bread
Coffee	Cream	Fruit Ice
Cream	Coffee or tea	Sugar
		Cream
		Butter
		Coffee or tea

Optional: use for children to include protein intake.
Omit if urine calcium is elevated in adults.

Summary of Diet Principles in Renal Stone Disease

Stone Chemistry	Nutrient Modification	Diet Ash (urinary pH)
Calcium	Low calcium (400 mg)	Acid ash
Phosphate	Low phosphorus (1000 - 1200 mg)	
Oxalate	Low oxalate	
Struvite	Low phosphorus (1000 - 1200 mg) (associated with urinary infections)	Acid ash
Uric acid	Low purine	Alkaline ash
Cystine	Low methionine	Alkaline ash

Adapted from Smith, D.R., Kolb, F.O., and Harper, H.A.: The management of cystinuria and cystine-stone disease. J Urol. 81:61, 1959

Reprinted with permission from Times Mirror/Mosby College Publishing, *Nutrition & Diet Therapy* by Sue Rodwell Williams, Ph.D., M.P.H, R.D., 5th Edition, 1985.

CHAPTER SIX

Water, Water Everywhere

E ven Hippocrates recognized the importance of drinking water. The practice of consuming large amounts of fluids has been recognized as an important factor in the prevention of kidney stones.

> The kidneys contain a nearly 40-mile network of tubes through which fluids filter. That's a lot of "freeways" for a kidney stone to get stuck in!

The kidneys process 100 gallons of blood a day, straining out waste via urine, then returning the purified fluid into the blood stream. That's why it is necessary to wash out these filtering tubes hourly.

An article in *The Canadian Medical Association Journal* (January 15, 1992) states that fluid intake is the most important dietary modification for patients with stones. It is the **only** dietary recommendation that applies to all forms of kidney stones regardless of the cause.

The *Journal* recommends that at least 8 oz. of fluid be taken with each meal, between each meal, before bedtime and when the patient gets up at night to urinate. This ensures that the fluid intake is spread out over the day and the urine never becomes concentrated. At least half this fluid should be taken as water. The rest is up to the individual, unless the diet is restricted in calcium or oxalate. In that case, overdependence on milk, tea, hot chocolate, draught beer and citrus juices must be decreased or avoided. Also important is that patients with ᵗones increase their fluid intake in hot weather and after ᴣorous exercise.

The average person loses six pints of water daily. Thus, rinking water helps accomplish this incredible cleansing ᵣrocess as well as helping to maintain the delicate water ᴊalance of the body.

Without Water—They're Back!

The tiniest portion or core of a living cell, called the nucleus, can form objects as large as stones only by growing itself or by combining with other nuclei to form a mass of relatively large clumps.

According to a revealing article by Fredrick L. Coe, M.D., Joan J. Parks, M.B.A., and John R. Asplin, M.D., published in *The New England Journal of Medicine* (October 15, 1992), these tiny cell cores cannot grow large enough to anchor and block off the kidney's tubular passages within the five to seven minutes it takes them to pass through the area where the kidney secretes urine.

However, they can form a collective mass within a minute and grow at leisure to stone size.

These collective masses must anchor themselves somehow in the kidney's system or be swept away in the urine when the patient drinks large amounts of water.

Kidneys At Work

Blood plasma processed in one day by the kidneys: 180 liters

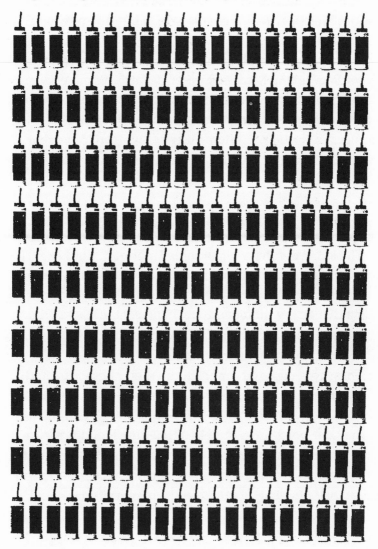

Total blood plasma in a typical person: 3 liters

Water and wastes excreted as urine (micturation): 1.5 liters

Reprinted with permission: FDR Publications, Allentown, Penn. 1993

Water is a simple prescription against a sea of health troubles. Author Kathryn Keller in her article "Water Works Wonders" writes that water can wash away the threat of a bladder infection, which is caused by a buildup of bacteria in the urinary tract.

According to Jean L. Fourcroy, M.D., Ph.D., a urologist at Walter Reed Army Medical Center in Washington, D.C., drinking plenty of water dilutes the concentration of bacteria and stimulates frequent urination which flushes out the microbes. In fact, Dr. Fourcroy advises women to prevent bacteria buildup by urinating every three to four hours during the day.

And All You Have to Do Is Micturate

The kidneys filter a remarkable amount of fluid each day— with minimum inconvenience to their owners. Sixty times a day, the body's blood plasma is processed by the kidneys. This means that at any moment, 20 to 25 percent of the heart's output goes to the kidneys. They receive about as much blood as the heart and brain combined!

These two organs do much more than filter waste and poisons from the blood. As the body's master chemists, they constantly balance the body's water and minerals, such as sodium and potassium, thereby regulating blood pressure. Thanks to the kidneys, the total amount of sodium in the body seldom varies by more than a few percentage points, even if you eat an entire bag of potato chips in one sitting.

The Cranberry Juice Miracle Cure—Or Is It?

Controlling urinary tract infections (UTI) is an important preventative measure since these infections are a risk factor in stone formation. Many patients are told to drink cranberry juice to prevent recurring urinary tract infections.

However, the latest research shows this to be on the fast track to becoming yet another old wive's tale.

Allan Bruckheim, M.D., a fellow of the American Academy of Family Physicians, and clinical associate professor of family medicine at New York Medical College in Valhalla, N.Y., wrote in his syndicated column that cranberry juice is no miracle cure. Yet many people drink glass after glass of cranberry juice, thinking it can cure bladder and other urinary tract infections.

Dr. Bruckheim points out that to understand the widely held idea that cranberry juice is an effective treatment for bladder infection, a word or two about urinary tract infections (UTI) is in order.

Women, he writes, are more susceptible to UTIs than men. It's estimated that one out of five women will suffer this painful and uncomfortable experience sometime during her lifetime.

The infection is signaled by a frequent urge to urinate. A burning sensation while urinating is almost always present. The infection is most commonly caused by a bacteria E. coli, which is normally present in the intestinal tract where it provokes no symptoms.

E. coli do not grow well in an acidic environment, and that forms the basis for the claim that cranberry juice can help. The theory is that, since cranberry juice in its undiluted form is not only acidic but bitter, it can cause the urine to become acidic enough to resist bacteria growth. An article in the *Journal of the American Medical Association* was also less than enthusiastic about the use of cranberry juice for controlling UTIs.

The present treatment for patients with such infections includes taking antibiotics and consuming lots of fluids to help flush the bacteria out of the system.

Sue Rodwell Williams, Ph.D., M.P.H., R.D., in her book *Nutrition and Diet Therapy* by Times Mirror/Mosby College Publishing, writes that commercially prepared cranberry juice is too diluted to be effective in acidifying the urine. Since juice from the grocery store contains only about 26 percent cranberry juice, a large amount would be required to achieve any consistent effectiveness as an urinary acidifying agent. Most physicians rely instead on drugs to obtain this effect.

Williams writes that some studies have indeed found significant decreases in mean pH with the use of cranberry juice. However, the concentrations and volumes of juice used in such studies are not practical for everyday use.

She concluded that general nutritional measures for UTI include acidifying the urine by taking vitamin C rather than cranberry juice, and drinking plenty of fluids to produce a dilute urine.

Give Me Water!

Health experts agree that people need to drink water even before they feel thirsty, particularly while dieting or exercising. According to Kathleen M. Cahill, a health and fitness editor who wrote the article "Lead a Course to Water" in *The Walking Magazine*, April/May 1988, new research shows that most people need to drink more water than they think—at least eight large glasses a day.

> A little more than two to three quarts or eight to twelve cups—is roughly what the "average" body uses and loses each day.

People who exercise regularly or live in a hot climate will need to drink even more than eight glasses daily to replace what they lose through excess sweat—as much as a quart or two more than usual. Experts advise that people should not wait until they're thirsty to drink; that's a signal they're already low on water. Juices, fruits, vegetables, and caffeine-free soft drinks can provide some of the daily water needed. But there's nothing better than plain old clear—and practically free—water.

Patients with kidney stones need to develop the habit of drinking lots of water—for the rest of their lives. When the urine becomes concentrated, the minerals it contains, normally dissolve, tend to solidify into everything from gravel to full-blown stones.

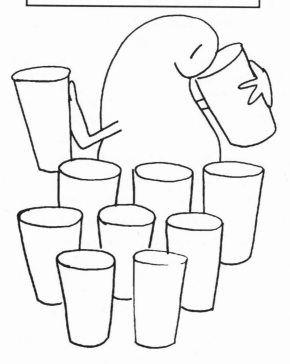

Sometimes half the day passes before one feels the need for fluids. No light goes on signaling: "time to drink water." How does one increase fluid intake?

Physicians and dieticians recommend that patients schedule time to drink glassfuls of water throughout the day. For example, drink a glass of water every hour in front of the computer at work and by day's end the daily requirement will be met.

Choose foods that contain high amounts of water—fruits and vegetables such as lettuce (96 percent), watermelon (93 percent), green beans (88 percent), broccoli (89 percent) and carrots (88 percent).

If plain water is boring, add a squeeze of lime, lemon or orange.

But I am Drinking Fluids!

Many patients who develop kidney stones *think* that as long as it's liquid, their beverage will benefit them. However, according to a study published in *Urology* (April 1992) by Gary H. Weiss, M.D., Ph.D., Patrick M. Sluss, Ph.D., and Charles A. Linke, M.D., cola-flavored carbonated beverages may actually enhance kidney stone formation.

Marked changes took place in the urine of patients who drank large quantities of cola-flavored carbonated beverages. These beverages possibly favor stone formation because of their high acid ash, high sugar, and/or high oxalate content.

The three participants who succeeded in drinking three quarts of cola per day showed an average of 8.3 mg. increase in their 24-hour urinary excretion of oxalate. Citrate (an inhibitor for kidney stones) decreased an average of 122 mg.

Coca-Cola® Says "Drink Me!"

While the test subjects were instructed to consume three quarts of Pepsi-Cola® per day for 48-hours, many people do not drink that amount in any one day. I contacted The Coca-Cola® Company regarding that study. Dr. Debra Ponder, manager for nutritional sciences said cola beverages have never been demonstrated in a controlled study to contribute to kidney stones.

She stated that one of the most recent and largest studies addressing this issue came from the Harvard School of Public Health. One of the researchers, Dr. Walter Willett, is internationally known for his studies on dietary intake as it relates to various disease states. This is the same study which found high dietary calcium intake decreased the risk of kidney stones.

The study found "no association between the consumption of sugared cola(s) and risk for kidney stones."

Even so, many doctors choose to be conservative in their recommendations to patients. If even a slight association exists between a particular disease and some dietary factor, patients are often advised to avoid that dietary food. With kidney stones however, one has to be careful when restricting fluids since dehydration is unquestionably linked to an increased risk for the development of kidney stones.

Most physicians tell their patients that coffee and caffeinated soft drinks are not good replacement fluids because the caffeine acts as a diuretic (increases the flow of urine) and causes even more loss of fluids. In addition to coffee and cola, tea and chocolate are common sources of caffeine and oxalates. The caffeine content in coffee depends on the variety of coffee bean and how it was ground and brewed. One cup of brewed coffee contains about 115 milligrams of caffeine. A cup of brewed tea contains about half as much. Soft drinks are a major caffeine source for children and adolescents because manufacturers often add caffeine to soft drinks. On average, caffeinated soft drinks supply about 45 mg. of caffeine per serving. A cup of hot chocolate contains only about 5 mg. of caffeine.

Alcohol, as anyone who has downed a beer or two can attest, has the same diuretic effect as coffee and colas containing caffeine. Alcohol may add to the risk of stone formation although the effects have not yet been extensively investigated. Recent evidence however suggests a correlation between alcohol consumption and levels of urinary calcium and uric acid. Beer (particularly draught beer) is known to contain oxalate and guanosine which is metabolized to uric acid in the body. Alcohol should therefore be consumed in moderation by people with calcium stones.

Dr. Sheldon Margen, a professor of public health at the University of California at Berkeley, and Dale A. Ogar, managing editor of the *UC Berkeley Wellness Letter*, in a published column in *The Times* titled "Water, Water—Every Day" wrote that water is considered the body's most essential nutrient.

For some patients with kidney stones, water may be the only way to prevent new stones from forming.

One gauge of whether you are in 'water balance' is to simply watch the color of your urine. If it is dark and yellow, you are not drinking enough. The urine should be pale and watery. It will have some color in the early morning due its concentration in the bladder, but during the day urine should be almost clear.

People who eat large amounts of protein each day require even more water to rid the body of dissolved breakdown products such as urea. Water helps dilute the food chemicals that cause stones to develop.

Again, water seems to be the best beverage! Here's a toast to Hippocrates!

CHAPTER SEVEN

The Urologist And The Patient

T he best time to choose a physician is when you don't need one. However, the first episode of an acute kidney stone attack often results in emergency room staff giving a referral to a physician the patient has never met.

Imagine getting married to someone immediately after you've been introduced! Having no time to get to know your bride or groom would bring much anxiety and little confidence. The relationship of physician to kidney stone patient may not be a marriage, but it is necessarily intimate and often long-lasting. It's satisfying only when trust and confidence are present. Establishing such a physician-patient relationship takes the time and effort of both physician and patient.

If you're satisfied with your doctor's competence, give the relationship time.

However, if your physician takes a 10-minute call from a colleague without apology while you've been telling him about your side pain, then can't remember what you were talking about, it's time to look for an empathetic, patient-centered physician.

If the physician looks at your chart without a word of greeting, then asks abruptly "what brings you here this time?" he or she might as well be waving a red flag: search for another physician!

Taking Part in Your Medical Care

While some physicians prefer an authoritarian, controlling approach, research suggests that may not be best. A study first published in *Diabetes Care*, then included in *The University of California Berkeley Wellness Letter* of April 1992, reported that diabetic patients trained to take part in medical decision making (specifically they received training in how to read medical records and how to question their doctors so that detailed conversations concerning their condition took place) were able to reduce their blood sugar more successfully than others.

The Berkeley Wellness Letter reported on other studies which "support the finding that patient involvement leads to better outcome in treating hypertension, ulcers, and other chronic diseases."

The article goes on to say, "American patients are entering an era of unprecedented sophistication and knowledge according to many observers. But do most doctors know that times have changed?"

The Berkeley Wellness Letter suggestions include :

■ Ask your doctor questions. One of your rights as a patient is access to information, including your medical records.

■ Patients must remember doctors are human, too, and often work under great pressure. Keep your remarks to the point. Before you go, give some thought to your concerns. If you're afraid of forgetting something, make a brief list.

- Be as well informed as possible.

- If you have a symptom you're uneasy about, don't put off mentioning it.

Locating a Specialist

The Consumer Guide provides excellent advice on choosing medical specialists. Often, as *The Consumer Guide* points out, patients are referred to specialists by their own family doctors or through other specialists. In fact, many specialists have a policy of not accepting a patient who has not first been examined and referred by a family doctor.

The reason for this, as *The Consumer Guide* explains, is that urologists deal exclusively with diseases and disorders of the urinary tract, the kidneys, the prostate gland and the male sex organs. The urologist has extensive knowledge of diagnostic procedures and surgical techniques, as well as the ability to treat infections of the urinary tract and the male reproductive system.

In selecting a specialist, you might follow your family doctor's advice, or the advice from the emergency room concerning follow-up treatment with a particular urologist.

If you know or suspect you need a urologist and have a specialist in mind, call the physician's office and ask what their policy is on seeing new patients.

Another way to find a specialist is through large teaching hospitals. In my area, a patient can make a self-referral to, for example, the University of California Davis Medical Center's general medicine clinic. That clinic would then make the referral to the urology department. The charge nurse at the

UCD's urology department explained this was "no problem and many patients were seen by outstanding specialists originating through self-referral."

Asking for a Second Opinion

You can always ask for a second opinion, as I have on occasion. Consulting with a second physician, after obtaining as much information as possible about your own or a family member's illness, gives you opportunity to find something that the first doctor may have missed. If both physicians agree, you'll gain greater confidence in the diagnosis and treatment.

A Harris poll conducted in 1987 found that 30 percent of all adults in the United States changed doctors because they felt their doctor was unwilling to talk to them—or unable to communicate in terms they could understand.

I can't stress enough the importance for patients who have kidney stones, or any other medical condition, to become as informed as possible about their medical condition.

The most compelling reason patients need to be as educated as possible about their own medical condition is because a correct diagnosis depends on it. According to an analysis by the American Society of Internal Medicine, correct diagnoses are 70 percent dependent on what patients tell their doctors.

Norman Cousins, author of the best-selling *Anatomy of an Illness* set out to prove that patients have the power, in partnership with their physicians, to make themselves well. In his book *Head First: The Biology of Hope*, Cousins wrote that nearly three out of four people he polled in the neighborhood surrounding the University of California at Los Angeles answered "yes" to the question: "Have you changed your physician in the past five years, or are you thinking of changing now?"

Most people changed physicians not for reasons of competence, but because of the doctor's manner. They were troubled by what they believed was insensitivity to their needs, or by the physician's lack of respect for their views.

Cousins supports the idea that having doctors and patients talk to one another is indispensable for an accurate diagnosis. This is a critical lesson for both physicians and patients to learn.

Using Medical Libraries as Research Tools

In most major cities large hospitals have medical libraries open to the public which provide a wealth of information via both consumer books and magazines, as well as established medical journals.

These consumer medical libraries are geared to the patient. While librarians are not there to provide medical diagnoses, they can guide you in the right direction for written articles and books and, in some cases, videos which will help you understand your illness.

I have used the most recent information I could find on kidney stones for this book from government materials, consumer libraries at hospitals and medical teaching centers. While materials can be obtained for a fee (in some cases a large fee), one can do medical research using both public libraries and consumer medical libraries at large hospitals for the price of a few dimes for the copy machine!

If one does not have time to research, a database search on a particular medical condition is worthwhile.

Some local city libraries (if they have not suffered drastic cutbacks) as well as university libraries may offer a medical database search which will scan hundreds of medical topics and provide the patient with a print-out of magazine articles for further reading (or re-searching as I like to call it).

Using Medical Data Bases

Until recently, only medical professionals and skilled computer users could tap into medical databases. One resource, the Health Reference Center, uses a hardware system made by Information Access in Foster City, California, to give consumers free use of a PC to locate and print out disease-specific articles.

Or, for a fee, a number of organizations will run computer searches on a medical topic and supply the results. Medical Information Service, operated by the nonprofit Palo Alto Medical Foundation (1-800-999-1999) is such a resource tool. Within 24 hours after a search request, MIS ships a bound report that includes up to 200 references and abstracts on a specific disease and a directory of support organizations. MIS gets a flat fee of $89 plus shipping per search, charging extra for actual copies of abstracted articles.

Other vendors include AIC Services in Ann Arbor, Michigan (313-996-5553) which charges $150 to $300, depending on the topic and how fast the search is delivered.

American Connection in Stanford, Connecticut, (203-359-9359) charges $300 to $500 for an exhaustive search that can take up to five days to arrive.

While these searches may provide a ton of information and assist you in becoming an informed patient, they are no substitute for necessary medical care.

Some physicians provide a portfolio of materials and booklets in their own offices. You may want to ask your urologist if he or she has any printed material about your own particular diagnosis.

The Need for Patient Education

Patients must become as educated as possible about their unique medical diagnosis. Many physicians may spend less than 10 minutes per office visit with a patient. In an article for *Stanford Medicine* (Winter 1985), Dr. Eugene Farber writes that physicians normally focus on diagnosis and treatment but rarely include guidance for prevention and self-help.

And you better start talking fast! According to an article in *American Health* (January/February 1987), you have an average of 18 seconds before your doctor will cut you off. According to Detroit internist Howard Beckman of Wayne State University, who analyzed tapes of 74 visits to seven doctors, only 16 patients were allowed to fully explain their problem. What's more, according to Dr. Beckman, doctors interrupted 52 patients before they'd even completed their first statement!

Dr. Beckman says some doctors interrupt for fear patients will talk forever. But his study showed that even the most outspoken patients need only about three minutes to speak their piece.

> Ask your doctor what you can do to prevent disease, and don't assume he or she will take the initiative. A survey of 322 adults from a small southern town found that although many wanted recommendations on preventative care, their doctors didn't automatically dispense them.
>
> *Health After 50*
> **The John Hopkins Medical Institutions**
> **February 1994**

Physicians don't intend to be callous, but they are indeed busy. I find it extremely helpful to bring a list of my questions, and I usually limit my list to six of the most important issues concerning my health during that visit.

Some questions I have asked my urologist included:

1. Will you spell the medical term for my metabolic disorder?

2. My research shows a diuretic may be helpful. Do you think I should take one, and if so, which one?

3. Could low potassium, as shown in my blood tests, be a reason why I feel tired?

4. Will I need another blood test in three months to monitor this new medication?

5. What is the difference between a sonagram and an x-ray in determining how many kidney stones I have? Do you feel one or the other, or even both, are necessary?

6. Living with a kidney stone that may pass at any time frightens me. How do I manage living with the fear?

7. What dietary guidelines can you recommend for me?

8. If I have lithotripsy, will it be necessary for me to have a shunt placed in my ureter? I'm afraid of that. What alternatives do you suggest? How can I cope with my fear of a shunt?

I believe informed patients who understand how to help themselves will enhance the effectiveness of office visits and treatment, saving both themselves and their physicians time, money and distress caused by the disease. I have learned no question is too stupid to ask and I have a right to demand answers.

"Current research has revealed that much of disease and illness may be preventable. Individuals are becoming increasingly aware of their health and are exercising some responsibility and control over it. We are making prevention a cross-cutting theme at Health and Human Services, building it into our programs and into our proposals for change. Across the board we are banking on prevention as the single greatest force."

—Richard Schweiker
Former U.S. Secretary of Health and
Human Services

Whose Medical Records Are They?

William Hafferty wrote in the April/May 1991 issue of *Modern Maturity* on unlocking your medical records. He stated that, "with the possible exception of a diary, it's hard to envision anything more personal and private than your medical records; yet a seemingly endless parade of folks may see them more easily than you can."

Knowing what is in your medical records, and thus knowing what is going on in your body, can make you a better informed, more involved patient. In addition, seeing your record will make you more attentive to your health and more in control of your health care. It helps establish a more open, equal, and therefore improved physician-patient relationship. It also protects your privacy by allowing you to inspect and correct information about you that will be released to others.

Obtaining your own medical records, especially regarding kidney stones, allows you to communicate intelligently with local medical personnel should an emergency arise.

I often enjoy taking short vacations to the rural coastline of Northern California. Many places I stay overnight are hundreds of miles from the nearest hospital facilities. To help me cope with the fear that I might have an acute kidney stone attack in "the middle of nowhere," my urologist gave me two things.

First, he gave me a prescription for pain medication with codeine. I bring this medicine on coastal trips and feel more confident, knowing I can manage the pain until I get to a hospital.

Secondly, I obtained my medical records in case I need a rural hospital's emergency room. I take my "passport"—my medical records—with me to avoid unnecessary medical tests or procedures.

Access to medical records varies from state to state. Currently there are 31 states with statutes granting patients rights to their medical records. The first step in obtaining your records is to simply ask your personal physician. If you are denied the records, request them in writing. If your health care provider won't give you your records, get the refusal in writing. From there your best bet is to contact a local patients' right group, or medical society.

Other resources are listed in **Chapter Ten— Resources: Beyond The Book**.

I paid $25 to obtain my medical records; the cost was a business decision made by my urologist. Paying this expense was necessary for me because I needed access to these records for peace of mind if not better health care.

The American Health Information Management Association (AHIMA) provides a free brochure on accessing your health records, titled "Your Health Information Belongs to You." When you need your records, the AHIMA suggests you contact the health information management or medical record department at the health care facility where you received treatment. This department will have a "release of information" person or office whose special responsibility is responding to requests for patient information.

To receive the AHIMA brochure, write to Professional Practice Division, American Health Information Management Association, 919 N. Michigan Avenue, Suite 1400, Chicago, IL 60611 or call (800) 621-6828.

One of the most outstanding books I have read is "*Medical Records: Getting Yours*" published by the Public Citizen's Health Research Group. Authors of the 1992 edition, Bruce Samuels and Sidney M. Wolfe, M.D., have written a consumer's guide to obtaining and understanding the medical record. The book includes a glossary of the most commonly used words found in medical records, as well as a state-by-state survey of legal laws on obtaining medical records.

Copies of the book may be purchased for $10 from Public Citizen's Health Research Group, Dept. MR2, 2000 P Street, N.W., Suite 700, Washington, D.C. 20036.

> A society that denies a person knowledge of his or her own state of health is toying with tyranny and is able to maintain this censorship only because in general the victims are weak, sick, alone and helpless.
>
> **—Ed Mulligan**
> **Medical Records Access Advocate**
> *Medical Records: Getting Yours*

Another source for help is the Grey Panthers, 2025 Pennsylvania Ave., NW, Suite 821, Washington, DC 20006 and the National Women's Health Network, 1325 G St. NW, Washington, DC 20005.

Equally important, knowing your family's history could save you a lot of pain, literally! Dan Maier, a spokesman for the American Medical Association, included this innovative idea in the AMA's 1992 list of "New Year's Resolutions for a Healthier America": write a family health history.

As reported in the January 27, 1992, issue of *Newsweek*, physicians have long been asking patients about their medical backgrounds. But many are amazed how few people know what their grandparents—or even their parents—died of and at what age. As scientists uncover hereditary links for more and more diseases, it is increasingly vital to learn what ailments lurk in family trees.

While I knew my mother, father and brother had kidney stones, until I wrote this book and started asking questions, I did not realize my paternal grandmother also had kidney stones! Maternal uncles and several cousins had also passed kidney stones. Had I known all this history, I might have avoided my painful predicament through prevention.

Assembling an ongoing health record for current family members can be a valuable legacy. I am educating my two children to make them aware of diseases that run in our family and how they may be able to prevent, or at least lessen the chances of certain metabolic disorders occurring. Foremost in their education is how and why kidney stones form and how they might be avoided.

Patients can find their way back to good health faster and stay there longer. Significant education is required for patients to be properly evaluated so preventive measures can begin before or with a first kidney stone—rather than after the pain and medical expense of additional stones!

CHAPTER EIGHT

Final Words on the Nuts and Bolts of Stone Prevention

For a child, the night-time fear of "monsters coming out of a closet" may be all too real. "Monsters" for me are the painful stones my body may produce unless I follow the preventative measures recommended by my urologist. Fortunately, new developments from the frontiers of medical research continue to offer kidney stone patients helpful information on preventing stones.

But what about the future?

Currently, funding for biomedical research is very tight and government programs for kidney stone research may be withering. The quarterly update from March 22, 1993 Urology Research Program of DKUHD Urolithiasis Research Grants reported total funding costs at $4,134,225.

However, in the same report, of the 14 R type grants which were funded, 10 terminated in the fiscal year 1993. While all of those researchers re-applied, they had not received favorable funding scores from either peer reviewers or multiple study section reviewers in 1993.

Kidney stone researchers received a little more than four cents per patient passing a kidney stone in 1993!

I believe we're worth more than that. We are experiencing an epidemic of kidney stones. Each year the patient numbers climb. It's time to stop this silent, yet painful suffering.

> Apart from the pain of renal colic, lost productivity, and other problems that recurrent episodes can cause, interventional procedures are still quite expensive—in the range of $5,000 to $10,000—compared with evaluation and preventive treatment. Comprehensive metabolic evaluation costs less than $1,000 a year and selective medical therapy less than $300 a year...specific medical therapy can prevent recurrence in more than 96 percent of patients.
>
> **—James E. Lingeman, MD**
> **—Glenn M. Preminger MD**
> **—David Wilson, MD**
> ***Patient Care*, September 30, 1990**

The Importance of Medical Tests

Even though lithotripsy and endourology have offered significant advances in the surgical treatment of renal stone disease, it must be remembered that these advances are helpful in 22 percent of patients requiring surgical intervention, and that 78 percent of patients do not require surgery, according to insurance information from StoneRisk Diagnostic

Profile. These advances do not address stone recurrence which continues to be a problem in up to 80 percent of all patients.

As I have previously written, keys to prevention and stone recurrence control begins with diagnostic work-up and medical management of the disease. According to the National Institute of Health Consensus Development Conference Statement on Prevention and Treatment of Kidney Stones, March 28-30, 1988, kidney stones recurrence can be prevented or controlled in 90 to 95 percent of patients with proper metabolic work-up and appropriate medical management which may include selective drug therapy.

A Diagnostic Profile

One test available to both physicians and their patients is a diagnostic profile. These series of monitoring tests have helped physicians diagnose and evaluate kidney stone patients. One profile is a urinalysis test panel which measures thirteen specific factors. In addition, the test calculates the risk for calcium oxalate, calcium phosphate, sodium urate, uric acid and struvite stones.

The test is convenient as patients can mail urine specimens directly from their home. For further details on the StoneRisk Diagnostic Profile contact Mission Pharmacal Company at 1(800) 531-3333. In Texas, call 1(800) 292-7364.

Stone-free Guidelines

The following general guidelines will discourage single-stone recurrences:

■ Increase fluids

Drink an 8-ounce glass of fluid (half of that water) each hour you are awake. If you awaken during the night to urinate, drink a glass of water. For most people, one glass during the night is enough.

The goal is to keep one's urine as light in color as possible. Increase the amount of urine to dilute and reduce incidence of crystals forming spontaneously. At first you may wonder if you can drink and process this much liquid. I've tried all kinds of tricks: adding lemon wedges to water, making sure I have a glass of water with me when I work at the computer, keeping a glass of water at my bedside during the night as well as nearby when I find time to read or watch TV. On days when I "free float" through my house, it's common for me to have several glasses of water in different locations. I find the more glasses of water I see, the more I am reminded to drink.

■ Diet

In susceptible people, certain foods may promote formation of kidney stones. Usually, the type of kidney stone you have will determine how to adjust your diet. You may be over-absorbing whatever it is your kidney stones are made of. For example, if you have calcium oxalate stones, you may have to adjust the foods rich in both calcium and oxalates. Or you might have to decrease dietary protein or sodium. Wash out these substances by drinking a lot of water!

- ■ Patients with renal hypercalciuria can be given a diet low in calcium with the addition of phosphate supplements.

- ■ Patients who are hyperuricosuric, often because of excessive purines from meat, poultry and fish, will need to reduce consumption of red meat, chicken, fish, dairy products, and oxalate-rich foods.

- Recurrent stones from patients with hypercalciuria while also increasing their fluids and eating a low-oxalate diet, may need a thiazide diuretic. If symptoms of gout develop, allopurinol may be prescribed.

- Recurrent stones formers with absorptive hypercalciuria will need increased fluid intake and a low calcium, sodium and oxalate diet and phosphate supplements.

- Patients with hyperuricosuria also need to increase their fluid intake; a diet low in purine and oxalate and moderate in calcium is recommended. If the patient finds it difficult to remain on such a diet, allopurinol may be prescribed.

- Your doctor and registered dietitian can help you tailor your diet. New dietary guidelines for patients with stones should be discussed with one's physician.

I keep lists of the foods high in oxalates and foods high in calcium (I copied the food list in the Nutrition Chapter) which I carry with me when I grocery shop. I don't necessarily look at my diet as restrictive—rather, I think of it as searching out foods which are positive and good for my overall health.

■ Avoiding Physical Changes in the Urine that May Lead to Stones

Physical changes in the urine that may cause susceptible persons to form stones include the following:

- Urine concentration: Many patients with kidney stones will hear their physicians tell them "Drink more water!" No use skirting the issue—many tests indicate if urine output is low.

■ Urine which is highly concentrated may result from a low water intake or from excess water loss, as in prolonged sweating, fever, vomiting, or diarrhea.

■ Additionally, urinary pH changes from its mean of 5.86 to 6.0 or more may be influenced by diet or altered by the ingestion of acid or alkali medications.

■ The Weather and Stones

Medical studies have pointed a finger at hot climates as accelerating stone formation because one is likely to lose more moisture through perspiration. I live in a very hot area of California: the Sacramento valley. I found it interesting that on the same hot July night that I rushed to the emergency room in dire crisis with a kidney stone, there were also two other patients being treated for the same condition! If I had a choice, avoiding hot weather—and hot locations—might have helped prevent my stone crisis.

■ Genetics

Kidney stones tend to run in families; whether it is actually a matter of genetics or common environmental factors such as diet or drinking water is not known. Because my paternal grandmother, my mother, my father, my brother and I all have kidney stones it seems likely they run in the family. However, my brother and I tend to form different stones; his are uric acid and mine are calcium oxalate.

■ Adding Dietary Fiber

The March 1992 issue of *Family Practice Recertification* on "Keeping Current in Gastroenterology" included an article on diet therapy to reduce kidney stone risk. The article recommended that dietary fiber, perhaps by binding calcium in the intestine and thus decreasing the intestinal transit time of calcium, may provide a means for reducing calcium absorption, particularly when combined with other dietary changes. Thus, supplemental dietary fiber, in addition to other modifications in diet, may be beneficial in reducing kidney stones.

The article also cautioned patients who are limiting their intake of calcium or oxalate to avoid milk, tea, hot chocolate, draught beer, and citrus juices.

RX: Lithotripsy in Most Cases, and a "Hammer" for Some

Physicians who met at the National Institutes of Health Consensus Development Conference stressed the value of preventative therapy. The physicians felt that the convenience and relative safety of lithotripsy (ESWL), as discussed in Chapter Four, may lead some patients to discount the importance of preventing new stones.

An article in the October 15, 1992 issue of *The New England Journal of Medicine* by Fredric L. Coe, M.D., Joan H. Parks, M.B.A., and John R. Asplin, M.D., reported that stones lodged in the ureter (above the pelvic brim) can be pushed upward into the renal pelvis. Lithotripsy, or ESWL, can be used, although pushing a stone backward requires cystoscopy (the insertion of an instrument that allows a visual examination) and the passage of a catheter up through the ureter.

Additionally, the use of a double-J stent (a urethral catheter shaped like a "J" at both ends) passed into the renal pelvis may improve the likelihood of completely removing the stone.

Today, in addition to shattering kidney stones with shock waves or pulsed laser light, urologists are testing a $6,000 to $10,000 device that does essentially the same thing as the more expensive lithotripsy machines. Urologist Stephen Dretler, MD and his colleagues at Massachusetts General Hospital in

Boston are testing the electromechancial impactor (EMI), a jackhammer-like device that can be threaded through the urinary tract to the ureter. Once it touches the kidney stone, the hammer is "fired" by an electrical pulse, and the hammering is repeated until the stone is shattered into fragments small enough to pass through the urine.

While kidney surgery may be needed if lithotripsy or other measures fail, most urologists perform this surgery only as a last resort.

Although recent concerns have been raised about stone fragments left behind by lithotripsy, the procedure is faster, simpler, safer and less costly than when major surgery was the only option. Currently, fewer than five percent of stone patients require surgery.

Prescriptions

Medications in the preventative course of kidney stones should not be overlooked. Uric acid stones may be dissolved by oral or injected medications.

Cystine stones can be treated with water and either the medications penicillamine or tiopronin. With either uric acid stones or cystine stones, treatment measures vary and the outcome may be poor if the stones are coated with calcium oxalate or struvite.

I have been taking Urocit-K, a potassium citrate product.

Other medications are appearing on the market. Potassium magnesium citrate is a new compound synthesized by Drs. C.Y. C. Pak, K. Koenig, R. Khan, S. Haynes and P. Padalino at the Center for Mineral Metabolism and Clinical Research, University of Texas Southwestern Medical Center, Dallas, Texas. Compared to a previous study focusing on potassium citrate, the newer potassium magnesium citrate was shown to cause a greater increase in urinary citrate. This medication also increased urinary magnesium which inhibits crystallization of calcium oxalate and uric acid in urine.

One can lessen the chances of a stone forming by taking certain medications carefully. For example, since overuse of calcium-containing antacids can cause stones to form, they should be used with caution.

Stone Prevention Clinics

If you have passed more than one stone, you may benefit from medical evaluation and preventative treatment of kidney stone disease in conjunction with your private physician or through one of several stone prevention clinics available throughout the United States. One such clinic, Stone Prevention Clinics of California, Inc. consists of a series of three office visits, appropriate laboratory and x-ray tests, and a yearly follow-up visit to evaluate the effectiveness of treatment. Studies to date suggest that 90 percent of patients with calcium oxalate stones (the most common type) who undergo treatment over a six-year period of time show no evidence of new stone formation.

While the clinic cannot guarantee the success of treatment (which depends to a large extent on the patient's cooperation), studies reveal new stones are prevented in the great majority of cases.

The Stone Prevention Clinic was established in 1988 to provide a medical adjunct to current surgical treatment of renal stones. The clinic has had a close association with the University of Chicago's Stone Prevention Program under the direction of Dr. Fredric Coe, a recognized pioneer in the field of kidney stone prevention.

Services provided include dietary consultation tailored to specific needs as well as "prevention before intervention," including access to an established university program.

Californians can get information on such clinics by writing Stone Prevention Clinics of California, Inc., 222 Oak Meadow Road, Los Gatos, California 95030, or calling (408) 374-1921.

Other referrals to stone prevention clinics throughout the United States may be obtained by calling the National Kidney Foundation office in your area. The national offices for each state are listed in the back of this book under **Resources— Beyond the Book**.

Checking Up on Your pH Levels

Drs. Joann LaPorte and Neil Baum, in the article "Kidney Stones: How to Identify the Cause and Prevent Recurrence" published in *Postgraduate Medicine*, April 1990, wrote that patients can monitor urine pH using nitrazine paper. I purchased a roll of nitrazine (or phenaphthazine paper) to monitor my pH levels. The dispenser has easy-to-read pH levels, coded by a color chart, and easy directions.

The paper helps me monitor my medication usage and often serves as an early warning if I miss a dose! I think of it as providing a psychological instant replay which shows how well I am doing with my medication. It's reassuring to know that some things do indeed work in this world!

The paper can be easily ordered from any pharmacy. I paid $27.87 for a five-yard roll. I can make the roll last longer by using shorter strips of paper. The supply will last for nearly four months.

Teaching Children—Prevention for Future Generations

I find it important, especially with my family's medical background, to stress the value of drinking large amounts of water to my own two children. They have watched me double over in pain from a traveling stone, and they have watched me recover from lithotripsy.

Just as it's important to teach children to cross the street safely, it's extremely important to teach children to drink water—especially when kidney stones run in the family.

My Own Bottom Line

As I finished researching and writing this book, I had a 15-month post-operative (due to the previous lithotripsy) exam with my urologist. You can imagine how wonderful it felt upon being told that I had no new kidney stones. While a small stone fragment remains from lithotripsy in my right kidney, that fragment showed no further increase in size! I have reached a sixteen-month anniversary free from the pain of kidney stones with no new stones!

In addition to the Urocit-K, I take magnesium supplements and vitamins B6, along with an all-purpose vitamin. I have also changed my diet to include more beans and rice for protein, while eating less meat and meat by-products. I've increased the amount of water I drink. I limit myself in drinking cola-flavored beverages, and have decided to continue limiting my calcium consumption upon the recommendation of my urologist. I've added more bran cereals to my diet.

The bottom line is that there is hope, and in many cases long-term prevention. Today, kidney stones don't have to recur.

CHAPTER 9

A Note to Kids Whose Parents Have Stones

—From a Kid Who Knows—

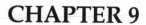

Hi! My name is Jennifer Golomb and I am the author's daughter. I thought it was important to have a "word" with kids who have a Mom or Dad who has kidney stones because it affects the whole family and it is scary to see your parent in a lot of pain. I am now 14 years-old.

I was 10 years old when my mom went to the hospital emergency room with a kidney stone. Until that time I never even knew what stones were, let alone know that we had kidneys. The closest thing I knew about kidneys was there was something named kidney beans and my brother loved to eat them, but to me they didn't smell too good.

When my mother had her first stone, I thought I was the one having a mid-life crisis, just like the adult game with that name. I thought I was the only kid in the universe with problems. From that time on, I was afraid that I would wake up one morning and my mom would be in the hospital again instead of at home taking care of me.

I was very scared and I felt very much alone.

My mom helped me put a smile on my face when two days after she had been to the emergency room she took me out to get my favorite ice cream in a waffle cone. She explained to me what stones were, how they leave the body and why there was so much pain, and what she could do to prevent new stones from forming. She said she thought she might even write a book about kidney stones! Even though I spent most of my time fishing out the biggest chocolate chip pieces I could find in the ice cream, her talk made me feel a lot better.

"Truth" is the hardest word in the English language, but it is the most important word to follow! Parents should always tell their children the truth when it comes to kidney stones.

Jennifer Golomb
Author's daughter

I love my mom and I usually know when something is wrong—if she is in pain or not feeling too well. I like to be told what I can do to help. If she has to go away to the hospital, I want to know what will happen to my brother and myself. The very, very most important thing for a parent to say is that "I will not die" from a kidney stone because that is the very first thing us kids think of. Also, tell your kid you love them.

Parents should let their children know that millions of children go through this experience each year with a parent. Kidney stones are a family experience and everyone needs to help.

Here is a list of some things a kid can do to help their parent:

1. You can put on a funny play for your parent to make them laugh.

2. Make a pretty get-well card.

3. You can clean up the house for your Mom or Dad. They don't feel well anyway and this is extra special to do.

4. Ask them if there is anything you can do, and if they want to sleep—let your Mom or Dad sleep.

5. When they feel better, make them a peanut butter and jelly sandwich (as long as that doesn't make another kidney stone!).

6. Bring them a glass of water to drink before they ask for one! In fact, bring them two glasses of water to drink!

7. Bring your parent a stone or a special rock from outside and make a joke out of it. You know—kidney *"stone."*

8. Go food shopping with your parent and take along the food chapter from my mom's book. Make sure your parent doesn't buy any foods which could make them form a new kidney stone. Find a new food to use instead of the "bad" food to eat.

9. It's important to take care of yourself, too, even if you are a kid because with some kidney stones, if your mom or dad has one, then someday you can get one! I try to drink lots of water. Teach this to your little brothers and sisters.

10. Most importantly, tell your parent how much you love them!

Good luck,
Jennifer

CHAPTER TEN

Resources: Beyond The Book

To request a Literature Search from the Kidney and Urologic Disease Subfile of the Combined Health Information Database (CHID) for topics in kidney and urologic diseases, contact:

National Kidney and Urologic Diseases Information Clearinghouse
Box NKUDIC
9000 Rockville Pike
Bethesda, Maryland 20892
(301) 468-6345

A current list of patient education materials as well as physician-related research articles on urinary stones is available, including the free brochure *"Prevention and Treatment of Kidney Stones."*

CHID is available on-line through BRS Information Technologies, a division of Maxwell Online, Inc. If you would like references to materials on other topics, you may request a special literature search of CHID from a library that subscribes to BRS or from the Information Clearinghouse. NIDDK is a service of the National Institute of Diabetes and Digestive and Kidney Diseases, National Institutes of Health.

The National Kidney Foundation, Inc.
Roster of Affiliates

National Kidney Foundation of Alabama, Inc.
1824 29th Ave., So. #216-C
Birmingham, AL 35209
(205)870-1112
(205) 870-1172 (Fax)
For All Mail:
P.O. Box 10101
Birmingham, AL 35202

National Kidney Foundation of Arizona, Inc.
4019 North 44th Street, Suite #201
Phoenix, AZ 85018
(602) 840-1644
(602) 840-2360 (Fax)

National Kidney Foundation of Arkansas, Inc.
4942 W. Markham, Suite 100
Little Rock, AR 72205
(501) 664-4343
For all mail:
P.O. Box 453
Little Rock, AR 72203

National Kidney Foundation of The National Capital Area, Inc.
2233 Wisconsin Ave., NW
Suite 320
Washington, DC 20007
(202) 337-6600
(202) 965-0517 (Fax)

National Kidney Foundation of Northern California, Inc.
553 Pilgrim Drive, Suite C
Foster City, CA 94404
(415) 349-5111
(415) 349-5115 (Fax)

National Kidney Foundation of Southern California, Inc.
5777 West Century Blvd., Suite 395
Los Angeles, CA 90045
(310) 641-8152
(310) 641-5246 (Fax)
(800) 747-5527

National Kidney Foundation of Colorado, Inc.
3801 E. Florida Avenue, Suite #503
Denver, CO 80210
(303) 759-5151
(303) 759-5162 (Fax)

National Kidney Foundation of The Delaware Valley, Inc.
325 Chestnut Street
Constitution Place, #904
Philadelphia, PA 91906
(215) 923-8611
(215) 923-2199 (Fax)

National Kidney Foundation of Florida, Inc.
625B No. Tamiami Trail
Nokomis, FL 34275
(813) 484-9597
(813) 484-0958 (Fax)
(800) 927-9659

National Kidney Foundation of Georgia, Inc.
1655 Tullie Circle, #111
Atlanta, GA 30329
(404) 248-1315
(404) 248-1320 (Fax)
(800) 633-2339

National Kidney Foundation of Hawaii, Inc.
Pacific Tower, #950
1001 Bishop St.
Honolulu, HI 96813
(808) 538-0104
(808) 523-3052 (Fax)

National Kidney Foundation of Illinois, Inc.
600 S. Federal, #403
Chicago, IL 60605
(312) 663-3103
(312) 663-5729 (Fax)

National Kidney Foundation of Indiana, Inc.
850 N. Meridian St., #203
Indianapolis, IN 46204-1108
(317) 693-6534
(317) 693-6538 (Fax)
(800) 382-9971

National Kidney Foundation of Iowa, Inc.
Executive Plaza
4403 First Ave., SE, #201
Cedar Rapids, IA 52402
(319) 393-8684
(319) 393-8791 (Fax)
(800) 444-8113

National Kidney Foundation of Kentucky, Inc.
250 E. Liberty St., #710
Louisville, KY 40202
(502) 585-5433
(502) 585-1445 (Fax)

National Kidney Foundation of Louisiana, Inc.
8200 Hampson, #425
New Orleans, LA 70118
(504) 861-4500
(504) 861-1976 (Fax)
(800) 462-3694

National Kidney Foundation of Maine, Inc.
169 Lancaster Street
Portland, ME 04101
(207) 772-7270
(800) 287-7270
For all mail:
P.O. Box 1134
Portland, ME 04104

National Kidney Foundation of Massachusetts, Inc.
180 Rustcraft Road
Dedham, MA 02026
(617) 326-7225
(617) 329-5074 (Fax)
(800) 542-4001

National Kidney Foundation of Michigan, Inc.
2350 So. Huron Parkway
Ann Arbor, MI 48104
(313) 971-2800
(313) 971-5655 (Fax)
(800) 482-1455

National Kidney Foundation of The Upper Midwest, Inc.
920 South 7th Street
Minneapolis, MN 55415
(612) 337-7300
(612) 337-7308 (Fax)

National Kidney Foundation of Mississippi, Inc.
2626 Southerland St.
Jackson, MS 39216
(601) 981-3611
(601) 981-3612 (Fax)
For all mail:
P.O. Box 55802
Jackson, MS 39296

National Kidney Foundation of Eastern Missouri & Metro-East, Inc.
3117 South Big Bend Blvd., Suite 200
St. Louis, MO 63143
(314) 647-9585
(314) 647-2644 (Fax)
(800) 489-9585
For all mail:
P.O. Box 430007
St. Louis, MO 63143

National Kidney Foundation of Nebraska, Inc.
2212 North 91st Plaza
Omaha, NE 68134
(402) 397-9234
(800) 642-1255

National Kidney Foundation of Nevada, Inc.
4100 Boulder Highway
Las Vegas, NV 89121
(702) 456-0026
(702) 457-1634 (Fax)

National Kidney Foundation of New Hampshire, Inc.
One Tremont Street
Concord, NH 03301
(603) 224-6641
(800) 354-3639

National Kidney Foundation of New Mexico, Inc.
1330 San Pedro NE, #103
Albuquerque, NM 87110
(505) 266-4573

National Kidney Foundation of Central New York, Inc.
731 James Street, #200
Syracuse, NY 13203
(315) 476-0311
(315) 476-3707 (Fax)

National Kidney Foundation of New York/New Jersey, Inc.
1250 Broadway, #2001
New York, NY 10001
(212) 629-9770
(212) 629-5652 (Fax)

National Kidney Foundation of Northeast New York, Inc.
23 Computer Drive E
Albany, NY 12205
(518) 458-9697
(518) 458-9690(Fax)

National Kidney Foundation of Upstate New York, Inc.
1 Grove Street, Suite 202A
Pittsford, NY 14534
(716) 264-0420
(716) 264-0109 (Fax)
(800) 724-9421

National Kidney Foundation of Western New York, Inc.
116 Linwood Avenue
Buffalo, NY 14209
(716) 882-2504
For all mail:
P.O. Box 651
Buffalo, NY 14209

National Kidney Foundation of North Carolina, Inc.
5970 Fairview Road
Three Fairview Plaza, #408
Charlotte, NC 28210
(704) 552-1351
(704) 552-7870 (Fax)
(800) 356-5362

National Kidney Foundation of Ohio, Inc.
1373 Grandview Ave., #200
Columbus, OH 43212-2804
(614) 481-4030
(614) 481-4038 (Fax)

National Kidney Foundation of Oklahoma, Inc.
5700 N. Portland, #317
Oklahoma City, OK 73112
(405) 947-6405

National Kidney Foundation of Oregon, Inc.
3689 SW Carman Drive
Lake Oswego, OR 97035
(503) 635-9977
(503) 697-3468 (Fax)
For all mail:
P.O. Box 222
Portland, OR 97207

National Kidney Foundation of Western Pennsylvania, Inc.
The Roosevelt Building
607 Penn Avenue, #205
Pittsburgh, PA 15222
(412) 261-4115, 16, 17
(412) 261-1405 (Fax)

National Kidney Foundation of South Carolina, Inc.
150 N. Ninth Street
West Columbia, SC 29169
(803) 796-5652
(800) 822-3216
For all mail:
P.O. Box 1316
Columbia, SC 29202

National Kidney Foundation of East Tennessee, Inc.
4450 Walker Blvd., #2
Knoxville, TN 37917
(615) 688-5481
(615) 688-0196 (Fax)

National Kidney Foundation of Middle Tennessee, Inc.
2120 Crestmoor Road
Nashville, TN 37215
(615) 383-3887

National Kidney Foundation of West Tennessee, Inc.
5545 Murray Road, #206
Memphis, TN 38119
(901) 683-6185
(800) 727-1039

National Kidney Foundation of Texas, Inc.
13500 Midway Road, #101
Dallas, TX 75244
(214) 934-8057
(214) 934-9357 (Fax)
(800) 441-1281

National Kidney Foundation of The Texas Coastal Bend, Inc.
3751 Up River Road
Corpus Christi, TX 78408
(512) 884-5892
(512) 884-2332 (Fax)
For all mail:
P.O. Box 9172
Corpus Christi, TX 78469

National Kidney Foundation of Southeast Texas, Inc.
1535 W. Loop South, #320
Houston, TX 77027
(713) 622-7440
(713) 622-8375 (Fax)

National Kidney Foundation of Utah, Inc.
Edgemont Professional Plaza
3707 N. Canyon Road, 1-D
Provo, UT 84604
(801) 226-5111
(801) 226-8278 (Fax)

National Kidney Foundation of Virginia, Inc.
503 Libbie Avenue, Suite C-2
Richmond, VA 23226
(804) 288-8342
(804) 282-7835 (Fax)

National Kidney Foundation of Washington
P.O. Box 84088
Seattle, WA 98124
(206) 322-7454
(206) 328-5074 (Fax)

National Kidney Foundation of Wisconsin, Inc.
7332 W. State Street
Wauwatosa, WI 53213
(414) 453-2830
(414) 453-2864 (Fax)
(800) 543-6393

For further information contact:
The National Kidney Foundation, Inc.
Affiliate Services Center
15 West Tenth Street, #1100
Kansas City, MO 64105
(816) 221-9559
(816) 221-7984 (Fax)
(800) 522-9559

The National Network of Libraries of Medicine
    The National Network of Libraries of Medicine (NN/LM)
provides health science practitioners, investigators, educators,
administrators, and patients in the United States with timely,
convenient access to biomedical and health care information
resources. The network is administered by the National Library of Medicine. It consists of 8 Regional Medical Libraries,
131 Resource Libraries (primarily at medical schools) and
some 3,300 Primary Access Libraries (primarily at hospitals).
Online access to MEDLINE and other databases are available .
The National Library of Medicine is part of the U.S. Department of Health and Human Services, Public Health Service of
the National Institutes of Health in Bethesda, Maryland 20894.
Each regional Library will direct you to a medical library or
libraries closest to your home.

The following is a list of the Regional Medical Libraries and the areas served by each.

Middle Atlantic Region
The New York Academy of Medicine
2 East 103rd Street
New York, NY 10029
(212) 876-8763
(212) 534-7042 (Fax)
States served: Delaware, New Jersey, New York, Pennsylvania

Southeastern/Atlantic Region
University of Maryland at Baltimore
Health Sciences Library
111 South Greene Street
Baltimore, MD 21201-1583
(301) 328-0099
(301) 328-0099
States served: Alabama, Florida, Georgia, Maryland, Mississippi, North Carolina, South Carolina, Tennessee, Virginia, West Virginia, the District of Columbia, Puerto Rico, and the U.S. Virgin Islands

Greater Midwest Region
University of Illinois at Chicago
Library of the Health Sciences
P.O. Box 7509
Chicago, IL 60680
(312) 996-2464
(312) 996-2226
States served: Iowa, Illinois, Indiana, Kentucky, Michigan, Minnesota, North Dakota, Ohio, South Dakota, and Wisconsin

Midcontinental Region
University of Nebraska Medical Center
Leon S. McGoogan Library of Medicine
600 South 42nd Street
Omaha, Nebraska 68198-6706
(402) 559-4326
(402) 559-5498 (Fax)
States served: Colorado, Kansas, Missouri, Nebraska, Utah,
and Wyoming

South Central Region
Houston Academy of Medicine-Texas Medical Center Library
1133 M.D. Anderson Boulevard
Houston, TX 77030
(713) 790-7053
(713) 790-7030 (Fax)
States served: Arkansas, Louisiana, New Mexico, Oklahoma,
and Texas

Pacific Northwest Region
University of Washington
Health Sciences Center Library, SB-55
Seattle, WA 98195
(206) 543-8262
(206) 543-2469 (Fax)
States served: Alaska, Idaho, Montana, Oregon, and
Washington

Pacific Southwest Region
University of California at Los Angeles
Louise Darling Biomedical Library
10833 Le Conte Avenue
Los Angeles, CA 90024-1798
(310) 825-1200
(310) 825-5389
States served: Arizona, California, Hawaii, Nevada, and U.S.
Territories in the Pacific Basin

New England Region
University of Connecticut Health Center
Lyman Maynard Stowe Library
263 Farmington Avenue
Farmington, CT 06034-4003
(203) 679-4500
(203) 679-4046
States served: Connecticut, Maine, Massachusetts, New
Hampshire, Rhode Island, and Vermont

For more information about specific
Network programs in your region, call
the Regional Medical Library in your
area at their direct number or dial
1-800-338-7657. This number is a toll-
free line for all Regional Medical
Libraries.

For general Network information contact:
National Network of Libraries of Medicine
National Library of Medicine
8600 Rockville Pike
Building 38, Room B1-E03
Bethesda, MD 20894
(301) 496-4777

For Information on Your Medical Records:
For a copy of the 69-page booklet *Medical Records: Getting Yours,* which provides information and advice on obtaining your medical records and includes a state-by-state survey of the laws governing patient access send $10 to:
Public Citizen's Health Research Group,
Publications Manager, Dept. MR2
2000 P St. NW, Ste 700
Washington, DC 20036.

For a copy of your Medical Information Bureau record (if one exists) contact:
MIB Information Office
PO Box 105 Essex Station
Boston, MA 02112
or call: (617) 426-3660)
Canadian residents contact: MIB Information Office
330 University Ave., Ste 102
Toronto, Ontario Canada M5G 1R7
or call: (416) 597-0590.

If you find an error, you can ask MIB to correct it.

A free brochure on "Your Health Information Belongs to You" is available by writing or calling the following:
American Health Information Management Association (AHIMA)
Professional Practice Division,
919 N. Michigan Avenue, Suite 1400,
Chicago, IL 60611.
(800) 621-6828.

For Referrals to Nutritionists:
As long as there is funding, you can get answers to your questions on nutrition—any time of the day. The toll-free Consumer Nutrition Hot Line (800) 366-1655, is provided by the National Center for Nutrition and Dietetics, the public-education branch of the American Dietetic Association. Registered dietitians are on the phone weekdays from 7 a.m. to 2 p.m. PDT. Or, you can call the same number and listen to a recorded message at any hour.

The Oxalosis and Hyperoxaluria Foundation
PO Box 1632
Kent, WA 98035
(916) 631-0386
An excellent support group for patients with oxalosis and hyperoxaluria, including a newsletter and dietary information.

Glossary

anesthesia	Produced in order to permit a painless surgical operation. Loss of sensation occurs.
anesthesiologist	a physician who specializes in the administration of anesthesia.
calcium oxalate	a chemical found normally in body tissues, including bone, blood plasma, etc.
calculus	a stone, such as a kidney stone or gall bladder stone.
cystitis	an inflammation of the bladder which is prevalent in women.
dehydration	the loss of water from the body. Such water loss can take place through the kidneys, the lungs, or perspiration.
extracorporeal shock-wave lithotripsy	this refers to lithotripsy, and is some times called ESWL.

hypercalcemia   a medical condition in which there are high levels of calcium in the blood, often leading to kidney stone formation.

hypercalciuria   a metabolic disorder which causes too much calcium to be absorbed from foods a patient eats.

hyperparathyroidism   excessive secretion of the parathyroid glands, producing a disease characterized by loss of calcium from the bones, often resulting in kidney stones.

hyperuricosuria   excess uric acid in the blood often resulting in gout, or kidney stones.

idiopathic   of unknown cause.

intravenous   within a vein. (An intravenous medication is one injected into a vein).

IVP   intra-venous pyelogram; x-rays taken after specific dyes have been given to outline the pelvis of the kidneys.

oxalate   a chemical.

oxaluria

having an excess of the chemical oxalates in the urine, sometimes associated with the formation of kidney stones.

lithotripsy

a medical procedure used to break up stones in the kidney and upper urinary tract. Lithotripsy uses shock waves generated outside the body to crumble the stone into tiny particles which are then passed out of the body in the urine.

predisposition

the state of being particularly susceptible to a certain condition or disease.

solute

a substance dissolved in another substance; to loosen.

spasm

an abrupt and forceful contraction of a muscle, usually maintained for several minutes or hours and frequently associated with marked pain.

struvite

an infection stone.

ureter

the tube leading from the kidney to the bladder.

uric acid	a normal chemical constituent of the blood. When present in excessive amounts it may be associated with gout or kidney stones comprised of uric acid. Uric acid is a product of purine, which is found primarily in animal protein.
urinalysis	examination of the urine
urine	the liquid excreted by the kidneys. Normally it has a clear amber color. It ordinarily contains urea, chlorides, and other chemicals. Urine does not normally contain sugar, albumin, pus, blood, bacteria, acetone or casts.
urogenital tract	the urinary and genital organs (kidney, ureter, bladder, prostate, penis, urethra, etc.).
urologist	a physician who specializes in diseases of the urogenital system.
UTI	urinary tract infection; recurrent UTI's may lead to kidney stones.

References

About Kidney Stones, *National Kidney Foundation Annual,* 1988.

"Are You Stone Prone?" *Good Housekeeping,* September 1989.

"Friendly, Interested, Respectful" *Berkeley Wellness Letter,* University of California at Berkeley, April 1992.

Betts, Kellyn S., Outpatient Lithotripsy: Simpler, Safer & Cheaper, *Medical Tribune,* March 17, 1988.

Brody, Jane E., Tiny Stones Inflict Goliath-sized Pain. *Contra Costa Times* July 16, 1992, p. 2E.

Bruckheim, Allan, M.D., Cranberry Juice No Miracle Cure, Health Column, *Sacramento Bee.*

Cerrato, Paul L., Nutrition Support-Kidney Stones Don't Have to Recur, *RN,* June 1992.

Coe, Fredric L., M.D., Parks, Joan H., M.B.A., Asplin, John R., M.D., The Pathogenesis and Treatment of Kidney Stones, review article, *The New England Journal of Medicine,* October 15, 1992.

Curhan, Gary C., M.D., Willett, Walter C., M.D., and others, A Prospective Study of Dietary Calcium and Other Nutrients and the Risk of Symptomatic Kidney Stones, *The New England Journal of Medicine*, March 25, 1993.

Clues to the Kidney Stone Mystery, *Science News*, September 28, 1985, p. 200.

Davis, Thomas Q., M.D., Is This Test Really Necessary?, *Modern Maturity*, February-March, 1987.

Ebisuno, S., M.D., et al. Results of Long-term Rice Bran Treatment on Stone Recurrence in Hypercalciuric Patients *British Journal of Urology*, March 1991; *Nutrition Research Newsletter*, June 1991. p. 71).

Farber, Eugene, M.D., Helping Patients Help Themselves, *Stanford Medicine*, Winter 1985.

Farley, Dixie, Vegetarian Diets: The Pluses and the Pitfalls, *FDA Consumer*, May 1992.

Getting Stoned on Protein, *Vegetarian Times*, January, 1992. p. 22.

Gutfield, Greg, et al. Fiber Power: Bran May Reduce Kidney-Stone Risk, *Prevention Magazine*, Feb. '91 p. 8.

Hafferty, William, "Whose Files Are They Anyway? Unlocking Your Health Records," *Modern Maturity*, April-May 1991. p. 68.

Harrison, Lloyd H., M.D. et al. Kidney Stones: New Treatments for an Old Problem, *Drug Therapy*, November 1988. p. 51.

Hunter, Beatrice Trum, Food for Though: Antinutrients, *Consumers' Research*, March 1991.

Iguchi, M.D., et al. Clinical Effects of Prophylactic Dietary Treatment on Renal Stones, *Journal of Urology* August 1990 (Diet and Kidney Stone Disease: Two Reports. *Nutrition Research Newsletter* November 1990, p. 128).

Jones, Wade Hampton. How to Find the Perfect Doctor., *Modern Maturity*, August-September 1989.

Kidney Stone Panel Stresses Long-Term Prevention, *Family Practice News*, Vol. 18, No. 11.

Kinder, Gentler Surgery, *Better Homes & Gardens*, September 1992.

Lake, Alice,. Taking the Pain Out of Kidney Stones and Gallstones, *Woman's Day*, September 13, 1988, p. 165.

Leadbetter, Guy W., M.D., et al. *Urology*. (Contempo '91 Special Issue: Reviews of Major Advances and Issues in Medical Specialties Over the Last Twelve Months) *The Journal of the American Medical Association* June 19, 1991. p. 3175.

Lemann, Jacob Jr., M.D., Composition of the Diet and Calcium Kidney Stones, an editorial, *The New England Journal of Medicine*, March 25, 1993.

Lerner, Seth P., M.D., Infection Stones, *The Journal of Urology* Vol, 141, March 1989. p. 753.

Lingeman, James E., M.D., Bioeffects of Extracorporeal Shock Wave Lithotripsy: A Worry or Not? *The Journal of Urology* September 1992. p. 1025.

Lingeman, James E., M.D. et al. Kidney Stones: Acute Management, *Patient Care,* August 15, 1990. p. 29.

Lithotripsy: A Shocking Approach to Urinary Tract Stones, *Hospital Practice,* July 15, 1986.

Magnesium Protects Against Kidney Stones, *Diet Counselor,* Special 1991 Edition. p. 11.

Mayo Clinic Health Letter Kidney Stones: How to Avoid Them, August 1992.

Meltzer, Jay I., Kidney Diseases, *The Columbia University College of Physicians & Surgeons Complete Home Medical Guide,* Edition 2, 1989. p. 650.

Motola, Jay A., M.D., Smith, Arthur D., M.D., Management of Upper Tract Calculi, *Urologic Clinics of North Ameria,* February 1990.

Paula, Tom, The Wave of Medicine's Future—Portable Operating Room Breaks Up Kidney Stones with Shock Waves, Longview, Washington *Daily News,* February 1, 1991.

Preminger, Glen M., M.D., Management of Nephrolithiasis and Ureterolithiasis, *Hospital Medicine,* January 1991, p. 22.

Preminger, Glen M., M.D., et al. Selective Medical Therapy of Renal Calculi, *Drug Therapy,* December 1988. p. 38.

Science Digest "Going After Stones" January 1980. p. 85.

Schmeck, Harold M. Jr., Kidney Stone Surgery Decreases, *The Sacramento Bee*, April 2, 1988, p. A18.

Sheinman, Allen J., Good News on Stones, *New Choices*, August 1989.

Sutter News Health Scene "Stone Crushing Comes to Sutter General Hospital" Spring 1988.

Toufexis, Anastasia. "The New Scoop on Vitamins" *Time Magazine*, April 6, 1992 p. 54.

Trouble with Kidney Therapy, *Sacramento Bee Final*, April 4, 1990.

United States Department of Health and Human Services, National Institute of Arthritis, Diabetes, & Digestive & Kidney Diseases Prevention and Treatment of Kidney Stones, NIH Publication No. 83-2495, August 1983.

Vitamin C: Probable Cause of Kidney Stones *The Journal of Urology*, 147 May, 1992 p. 1215.

Wasco, James M.D., When—And How—To Get a Second Opinion, *Woman's Day*, July 26, 1988. p. 14.

Wasserstein, Alan G., M.D., Kidney Stones: Advice on Preventing First Episodes and Recurrences, *Consultant*, May 1986. p. 81.

Wagner, Mary. "Jackhammer Could Crush Cost of Treating Kidney Stones." *Modern Healthcare,* June 10, 1991 p. 19.

Weiss, Gary H. M.D., Ph.D., et al. Changes in Urinary Magnesium, Citrate, and Oxalate Levels Due to Cola Consumption. *Urology* April 1992. p. 331.

Wilson, Tad W., M.D., and Preminger, Glenn M., M.D., Extracorporeal Shock Wave lithotripsy: An Update, *Urologic Clinics of North Ameria,* February 1990.

"Kidney Stones," *Patient Care,* August 15, 1990.

University of California at Berkeley Wellness Letter "Ask the Experts: Will Taking Vitamin B-6 or magnesium prevent kidney stones?" September 1991.

University of California at Berkeley Wellness Letter, "Fascinating Facts," March 1992.

Index

medical data base 114
medical evaluation 9, 129
Medical Information Service 114
medical libraries vii, 68, 113,
    148, 149, 151
medical records 110, 117–120,
    152, 183
Medical Records: Getting Yours
    119, 152
medical therapy 35, 122, 162
medication. *See* kidney stones
men iii, 1, 2, 13-14, 16, 20, 26,
    29, 34, 38, 41, 72-74, 76-
    78, 103, 111
metabolic abnormalities 35, 78
metabolic disorder 17, 20, 26,
    42, 116, 120, 156
metabolic disturbance 17
metabolic evaluation 122
metabolism 15, 27, 40
methionine 42, 96, 98
micturition 34
milk 36-37, 72-73, 84, 88, 90-91,
    93-97, 100, 127. *See also* dairy
    product
mineral deposit 15
minerals 21, 26, 34, 102, 105
Modern Healthcare 58
Modern Maturity 117, 160-161
Mulligan, Ed 119

N

Nakagawa, Yasushi 16
National Institute of Health 123
National Kidney and Urologic
    Diseases Information 137
National Kidney Foundation, Inc.
    Roster of Affiliation 138
National Kidney Foundation, The
    2, 85, 130, 138
National Network of Libraries of
    Medicine 148
National Women's Health
    Network 120
nausea 1-3, 6-7, 50-51, 68

New Choices 62, 163
New England Journal of Medicine
    72-73, 76, 100, 127, 159-161
Newsweek 120
nitrazine paper 130
Northern California Kidney Stone
    Center 51
nutrients 71, 71–72, 80-81, 160
nutrition v-vi, 11, 68, 69–86,
    104, 107, 153, 159
Nutrition & Diet Therapy 98
Nutrition Desk Reference 81
Nutrition Research Newsletter 78-
    79, 160-161

O

obesity 49
O'Brien, Walter M., M.D. 28
occupation. *See* kidney stones
Ogar, Dale A. 108
omega-3 fatty acids 71
orange juice 23, 89, 97
organic substances 24
osteoporosis 73, 74, 82, 84
oxalate 18, 21-22, 25, 35-38,
    70-73, 75-77, 79-80, 83, 84,
    87, 98, 100, 106-108, 124-
    125, 127, 156-157, 164

P

Pahira, John J., M.D. 28
pain. *See* kidney stones
Palo Alto Medical Foundation 114
parathyroid glands 28, 156
Patient Care 35, 122, 162, 164
patient education v, 11, 115, 137
Pechter, Kerry 80
penicillamine 42, 128
peptic ulcers 36
pH levels 130
phosphorus food 37
physical malformation 49

strainer 10, 11, 54, 66
struvite vi, 15, 20, 31, 32, 40,
    41, 90-91, 98, 123, 128, 157
supplements 23, 37, 74, 80-81,
    85, 124-125, 131
surgery i, 5, 8, 9, 46-50, 56,
    68, 122, 128, 161, 163
Sutton, Roger A.L., M.D. 26
sweating 20, 126
symptoms. *See* kidney stones

T

tea 36, 70-72, 84, 88-91, 94, 96-
    97, 100, 107, 127
Tennessee 29, 146, 149
testosterone 14
tests 3, 5, 8-9, 17, 21, 46, 49,
    62, 83, 116, 118, 122–123,
    125, 129. *See also* blood; urine
thiazides 82
Thiola 42
Thun, Michael 29
tiopronin 128
toxic substances 22, 30
trace elements 28
tranquilizer 50, 63-64
trauma 3, 22
treatment. *See* kidney stones
Trinchieri, A., M.D. 78
triple-phosphate stone 40
tubes 32, 34, 99
tumor 28, 58

U

ultrasonic 45, 58
ultrasound 49
United States, southeast 28
University of California Davis
    Medical Center 48, 111
urease stone 40
ureteroscope 58
ureters 9-10, 32, 34-35, 54, 58
urethra 32, 34, 46, 127, 158
uric acid vi, 17, 21, 23, 27, 31, 38-
    40, 74, 77-78, 94, 98, 108,
    123, 126, 128-129, 156, 158

urinalysis 49, 123, 158
urinary infection 7
urinary stones i, 28, 35, 137
urinary system 32, 35, 49
urinary tract 1, 18, 24, 27, 30,
    32, 51, 58, 102, 111, 128, 157, 162
urinary tract infection
    22, 40, 43, 90, 102-103, 158
urinary tract obstruction 20, 32
urine 3, 7, 9-10, 15-16, 21-23, 25-
    29, 32, 34-36, 39-42, 48-49,
    51, 54, 62, 65-67, 71, 74-77,
    80, 83, 85, 97, 99-101, 103-
    108, 123-126, 129, 157, 158
urine pH 27, 40, 74, 77, 98,
    126, 130
Urocit-K 128, 131
urologist v, vii, 12, 21, 25, 50, 60-
    63, 66, 71-72, 102, 109, 121,
    127-128, 131, 158, 178
Urology 106, 161, 164

V

vegetarian 25, 76-77, 97, 160
Vegetarian Times 76, 160
vitamin A 21
vitamin B6 37, 80-81, 85, 131
vitamin C 21-23, 37, 39,
    85, 104, 163
vitamin D 21, 28, 36, 82, 85
vitamins 79, 81, 85, 163

W

Walking Magazine, The 104
Wasserstein, Alan, M.D. 15, 80,
    163
waste 34, 99, 101, 102
water 21, 25-26, 28, 34, 36-37,
    42, 47-48, 50-51, 54-55, 59, 65-
    66, 79, 85, 88-89, 99, 101, 124-
    126, 128, 131, 135, 155
Weiss, Gary H., M.D., Ph.D.
    106, 164
Wellness Letter
    70, 108, 110, 159, 164
Willet, Walter, M.D. 107, 160

Send a Copy of This Book to a Friend

You may know a person or two, among all your friends and relatives, who is in need of information found in this book. Someone who could benefit and appreciate receiving a copy.

For additional copies we suggest you first try your local bookstores. But, if they happen to be out of stock, we will be pleased to receive your order directly, and it will be shipped immediately. Just drop a letter with your name and address, and check or money order for each book purchased. The price is $12.95 plus $2.50 postage and handling (California residents add appropriate sales tax).

Send to:
Four Geez Press
1911 Douglas Blvd., Suite 85-131
Roseville, CA 95661